PARTICIPATION IN HEALTH

Participation in Health

J. McEWEN, C.J.M. MARTINI and N. WILKINS

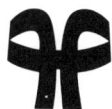

CROOM HELM
London & Canberra

© 1983 J. McEwen, C.J.M. Martini and N. Wilkins
Croom Helm Ltd, Provident House, Burrell Row,
Beckenham, Kent BR3 1AT

British Library Cataloguing in Publication Data

McEwen, J.
    Participation in health.
    1. Health education
    I. Title
    613'.07   RA440

    ISBN 0−7099−1754−6

Printed and bound in Great Britain by
Biddles Ltd, Guildford and King's Lynn

CONTENTS

TABLES AND FIGURES

Tables

Figures

PREFACE

The authors are indebted to the Health Education Council for the financial help which made this review possible and to Ms Rochelle Bock who worked with us as a research assistant during the search and collation of the literature. We would express our thanks to Mrs Judy Rose for her work in preparing the manuscript. We are grateful for the information, advice and help given to us by staff involved in various research projects, individuals and members of self-help organizations. For deficiencies we alone are responsible.

It is hoped that this review will be of interest to those concerned to promote participation in health and that it will provide a stimulus for further research and the establishment of innovative research projects.

PARTICIPATION IN HEALTH

Chapter One

INTRODUCTION

"In the art of medicine, there are three factors -the disease, the patient and the doctor. The doctor is a servant of the art. The patient must co-operate in fighting the disease." When Hippocrates wrote those words over 2000 years ago, he recognised the importance of active participation by patients in their own health care although some physicians and patients may not have shared his views. Like most controversial subjects, there is a need for regular review in the light of changing scientific knowledge, public attitudes and professional opinion. We believe that the subject of this book is likely to be one of the major determinants of the health of our communities and the type of care that will be provided. While we make no claim that we have covered all aspects of participation, we hope that some of the points that we raise and the illustrative examples will stimulate discussion.

'Self-help', 'consumer participation' and 'demystification' are terms now found regularly in both professional and lay literature. They are part of an amorphous and yet manifest social phenomenon which embraces such notions as self-care, alternative medicine, consumer satisfaction, holistic medicine and patient power. Many of these terms mean different things to different people; many have emotive connotations and no single term describes comprehensively the movement that is so widespread at present. Accordingly we have preferred to use the term 'participation' to examine the process whereby a person can function on his or her own behalf in the maintenance and promotion of health, the prevention of disease, the detection, treatment and care of illness and the restoration of health or where recovery is not possible, adaptation to continuing disability. This may occur both

1

independently of, or within, the existing system of care. We also intend the term 'participate' to include activities performed by an individual on behalf of others in areas of health care similar to those just outlined and in the planning, management and evaluation of health care provision.

We consider that the main concepts involved in this participation consist of: firstly, an active involvement by the individual in all aspects of his or her own health care rather than the traditional passive role normally associated with being a patient ('self-help'); secondly, a process of substitution and/or complementation whereby tasks normally thought to fall within the medical or professional sphere are taken on by the individual ('demedicalisation' or 'deprofessionalisation') and thirdly a desire to assume responsibility for decision making with regard to the wider aspects of social policy and health care provision ('democrat-isation').

To some health professionals these developments are threatening; to others they seem irrelevant or a matter for scorn and while some lay people enthusiastically support these ideas, others are happy to rely on professional help and fear the implied responsibility or possible difficulty in obtaining professional help. Frequently the arguments are blurred by the emotive language of the proponent or obscured by jargon.

This book will attempt to describe the present 'state of the art' by examining the rhetoric, reviewing the existing literature and studies, indicating the lack of evaluative research and will seek to produce a synthesis of the movements that are currently being actively pursued by many enthusiasts. Although much has been written in favour of these approaches, mention will also be made of the possible risks. As the field is uneven and does not have clear boundaries, it is impossible, in the limited scope of this study to be comprehensive, but rather the aim will be to illustrate the trends from the huge and rapidly expanding field of literature and, by clarifying the underlying theoretical concepts, to devise strategies for further intervention programmes and evaluative studies.

The Social Context
The whole issue of participation must be seen initially in the historical context. Is this something completely new in the health field or has

it a long tradition? This question is closely
related to social change, new patterns of health and
illness and the changing role of medicine and the
medical profession. The question of participation in
health is inevitably linked with the wide political
issues of participation in other areas of life such
as industry, education, housing and environment.

A Reaction Against Present Services?
How much does the current movement represent a real
desire to participate meaningfully in health
decisions or how much does it reflect a criticism of
the quality and quantity of the professional
services? Is it a logical extension of existing and
widely practised self-care, as, for example, is
evidenced, by the extensive use of self-medication,
or is it a wish to experiment with new forms of
health care, either based on alternative
philosophies or derived from the expertise of those
who themselves experience the problem? Is the aim to
set up an alternative to existing services or to work
with them and to provide different or additional
skills, care or advice?

The Place Of Health Education
We are not concerned primarily with the entire fields
of traditional health education or preventive
medicine, but aspects of these important disciplines
will be discussed. The contribution and influence of
the mass media is such an enormous, complex and
controversial topic that it cannot be considered
fully. The objectives and methods of health
education, and their relevance to participation will
be examined: the different approaches and their
application to different target populations;
education for health attainment and maintenance, for
self-diagnosis, medication and help with specific
problems; education for participation and better
utilisation of health resources. These illustrate
the breadth of the subject.

State, Professional And Consumer Perspectives
Some of the possible roles and contributions of
government, professionals and consumers will be
discussed. Illustrative material will be drawn
primarily from Britain, but examples of new
approaches from other countries will be included. New
legal and ethical responsibilities must be
considered.

Advantages And Risks

Do the possible advantages outweigh the possible risks? The advantages may consist of: increased patient responsibility and commitment to health and health promoting activities; the contribution of new community based resources; the development of a new ecological concept of health; an improved integration of existing health services combined with better utilisation. While the risks may include: possible increased delay in seeking care; ill-effects of self-diagnosis and self-medication; risks of conflicting advice; the danger of uncontrolled and unevaluated treatment; the misuse of highly technical information and the alienation of professionals. These must be compared with the advantages and the risks of the present system.

Doctor-patient Relationships

Issues such as these have implications for patient-professional relationships. They require that we re-examine the team concept and the roles of the different professionals involved in health care. This in turn necessitates a review of the whole field of education of professionals. From such a re-examination, is it possible to see the way to the development of a needs-derived approach to health, health planning and evaluation of health care, associated with the determination of priorities and allocation of resources to meet these needs?

This is too large and too important an area to continue to mushroom without efforts at evaluation and attempts to relate it either to the health and social needs of individuals and communities or to existing services both professional and other. It is our view that the implications for the health professional and the public are enormous and as yet not clearly understood; it is however an appropriate time to begin to examine them.

Chapter Two

A NEW PERSPECTIVE?

"None practise physic nor professeth midwifery but charitably one neighbour helpeth another". This old quotation(1) clearly indicates the simple approach to health that was common in many rural communities. Although physicians, surgeons and women with experience in midwifery existed, many people in the country areas were dependent on the limited resources of the particular community. Self-help and professional services existed together, their use and availability depending on finance, custom and situation.

Woodward and Richards (2) describe the significance of Popular Medicine and Health Care in Nineteenth Century England. Closely linked with the traditional folk medicine and the mutual self-help, there was an extensive publishing business. Books and pamphlets on all aspects of health existed. They were generally extremely practical, ranging from comprehensive encyclopaedias to small pamphlets on individual topics. They included both prevention and cure, they covered diagnosis, treatment, convalescence and rehabilitation, and ranged into many aspects of household management. Many were closely related to the various religious movements of the nineteenth century, with an holistic approach to physical, mental, social and spiritual well-being.

In the Prefatory Note to one such publication of 1890 (3) it is stated that:

the diffusion of sound information, in a popular and readable form, fitted to make the people sensible of their responsibility, and lead them to use all the means in their power to preserve their own health and the health of those dependent upon them, so that they may be able to fulfil in the best manner, all the purposes

of their existence, is therefore one important
branch of the work of THE RELIGIOUS TRACT
SOCIETY.

It included chapters on such issues as 'How to
avoid dying before the time', 'Blood Poisons', 'On
the care of children' and 'How to be healthy in one
room'.
This exemplifies the other type of self-help
that was common in the nineteenth century. The self-
help of Samuel Smiles (4) was based on personal
initiative, hard work and dedication and individuals
were to overcome all problems and adversity by their
own efforts.
Unfortunately it is not possible in this review
to trace the developments in philosphy, social policy
and service provision that have taken place since the
latter part of the nineteenth century; but it has
been documented elsewhere how the medical profession
gradually increased in knowledge and power and the
health services became more comprehensive and freely
available (5). The emphasis switched to the
effective prevention of disease and the competent
treatment of a large range of conditions. However, as
will be seen, when we discuss primary care, there is
a considerable departure from health (6) that is
never brought to any health professional and the
practice of self-medication is widespread. What is
perhaps remarkable is not that most people treat
themselves, but that this should be commented upon.
Currently the issues outlined in the
introduction are matters of concern in both the
developed and developing countries.

WHY NOW?

Why is participation confronting us now? Why is it a
topic for debate in the 1980's? These questions
relate not only to the field of health, but to all
aspects of social life. Many factors and a number of
different trends have contributed to the present
position. The most important of these are outlined
here:-

The Changing Patterns Of Health And Illness
The Public Health Movement which developed from the
pioneering work of Chadwick (7) and other reformers
of the last century, using the skills of preventive
medicine, bacteriology, engineering and health

education was extremely effective in reducing the
mass communicable diseases. (5) This was followed by
more direct therapeutic intervention in this
century, resulting in the possibility of rapid and
usually complete recovery from acute illness.
However, perhaps the greatest contribution to
improved health status resulted from changes in
housing, nutrition, education and other social
changes in the 19th and early 20th centuries.

This facility to prevent and treat communicable
and acute illness has both increased, and made more
apparent, the existence of a variety of more chronic
conditions. (8-11) This well monitored shift from
acute to chronic illness is one factor in the rise of
patient participation. Unlike the former, the latter
has characteristics making self-help appropriate;
namely, incurability, an emphasis on the need for
continuing care and some degree of chronic
impairment, but the possibility of a viable lifestyle
if rehabilitative procedures are followed.

These features provide sufficient hardship to
give sufferers and relatives motivation and a bond,
with demonstrable room for improvement in the
management of the condition, so that group activities
can provide real practical help and emotional
support.

The prime example is chronic degenerative
disease such as ischaemic heart disease or stroke.
There is an increase in conditions of disability
resulting from the contribution of sophisticated
medical technology which can intervene in a disease
process to prevent death but not necessarily to
produce cure. This is also seen in conditions such as
renal failure and severe head injury. Similarly
there is an increase in, and increasing recognition
of, less severe but nonetheless incapacitating
conditions such as the psycho-social problems.

New areas of uncertainty exist - there are
problems of definition - what is health, what is
illness, what is normal, what is deviance? (12-19)
'Stress' (20-23) is discussed by both patients and
professionals, assumptions are made about its nature
and its effects, and the pharmaceutical industries
spend much of their time producing drugs to alleviate
the results of these problems. And yet it remains
difficult to measure it and to know at what stage it
becomes pathological.

Some of these physical, mental and social
problems are of great severity, others are less
dramatic but nevertheless cause considerable disability, hardship, suffering and inconvenience both

to individuals and those closely associated with them. (24) Many of these conditions have a behavioural component both with regard to aetiology and to continuing care and support. Patients are having to live and work (25) with conditions which leave a greater or lesser degree of handicap and often require long term care and support from a variety of professionals and individuals in the community. Indeed, many would agree with Illich (26) that these problems have become too medicalised and that new approaches (27) not based on a professional approach or the traditional medical model are required in both prevention and care.

The Health Care System

Thirty years after the introduction of the National Health Service in Britain, there is an increasing awareness of some of the dilemmas that beset such an enormous complex organisation. The fact that the problems in such a service are closely linked to the structure of society, and that the way in which the service develops over the next 30 years depends on the way in which British society evolves, is clearly stated by Klein: (28)

> For, in many respects, the NHS's problems now illustrate - if in a particularly florid form - the problems of British society. Its institutional structure reflects an attempt to reconcile three potentially conflicting aims of policy: to accommodate the demands for national policies designed to share out scarce resources in a fair and rational way; for participation in decision-making by those actually working in the organisation; and for responsiveness to the views of the users of the service at the point of delivery. In all these respects the NHS reflects some general trends. Firstly, there is a widespread consensus that social policies should be egalitarian in intent: that there should be national policies for the distribution and use of resources. Secondly, there is a widespread acceptance that - whether in the social services or in industry - the trend is towards greater participation for workers in decision-making. Finally, there is general support for greater consumer part-icipation.

As Klein points out, however, the attempt to reconcile these various aims can develop into a 'stale-mate' situation. Implementation of national policies requires centralised control. But effective participation by either workers or consumers, necessitates flexibility, local democracy and diffusion of control. And so in-built into the system is both the facility of the centralised power to create policy and the facility of the staff and recipients to reject it.

The Limitations of Modern Medicine

The theme has been graphically tackled by a number of writers. Carlson (27) speaks of the 'end of medicine', while Illich (26) writes of the medical establishment as a 'major threat to health'. This is part of the wider issue which has been called 'the crisis of contemporary professionalism'. There is criticism of the bureaucracy, the inflexibility and the impersonal nature of the service, combined with the recognition that medicine has limitations and cannot cure every ill. (29) There is a realisation that much of the improved health over the last century is the result of improved socio-economic conditions, improved nutrition, better housing and an adequate supply of pure water and an efficient sewage system. Health services have made a limited contribution to health. (30) The risks of modern medicine as well as the advantages are also better known.

Iatrogenesis has grown to such proportions that it can no longer be ignored. Estimates differ but certainly some of the patients being treated today would not be ill if they had not been treated yesterday. (31-33) It is doubtful whether this message has filtered through to many consumers who still want a prescription for the most minor complaint or to many doctors who are willing to collude with such expectations.

For those who consider that they have suffered badly at the hands of the medical profession - the vaccine-damaged children, the thalidomide babies, the DES-Watch daughters of the United States of America (young women suffering vaginal cancer because of drugs administered when they were in utero) - self-help groups seem to be the only answer since they feel that they cannot put their trust in the professionals again.

As for the mistakes which occur in health services, the only answer it is argued, is for the

patient to be fully involved in the decision-making
process - only the patient cares enough about the
outcome to check and double-check.

The Growth Of The Consumer Movement
This movement has been seen in most countries
although its exact nature has varied. Writing about
the United States of America, Perlman (34) summaries
the main changes:

> Whereas in the 1930's struggles for social
> change took place for the most part at the point
> of production, with the lines of conflict drawn
> between workers and management, and the union
> movement playing a prominent progressive role,
> today's progressive struggles are often waged
> at the point of consumption. Given the greatly
> expanded role of the state, more and more such
> conflicts are between individuals or groups of
> individuals and the state or some part of its
> regulatory or delivery apparatus. The seventies
> are spawning a plethora of grassroots
> associations involving local people mobilized
> on their own behalf around concrete issues of
> importance in their communities. An outgrowth
> of the social movements of the past 15 years,
> yet vastly different in organization and style
> from the media-attracting demonstration and
> protests of the sixties, the new grassroots
> activity is emerging at a time when the fund-
> amental values and institutions of this country
> have been severely undermined and their legit-
> imacy called into question.

Perlman characterises the social movements of
the sixties as mass movements mobilizing around a
variety of national issues. The civil rights
movement, the welfare rights movement, the anti-war
movement, the women's movement, the ecology movement
- all challenged basic assumptions about the way
their country was governed and demanded changes in
national policies.

The seventies' movements, however, Perlman
perceives as grassroots associations springing up
out of disillusionment with the ability of government
to improve the lot of ordinary people. This
pessimism grew with a series of national and
international events which shook peoples' faith in
the state: Watergate, the ending and aftermath of the
Vietnam war, the challenge to the hegemony of the

American economy by other countries and the discrediting of the intelligence agencies.

All this has led to people feeling the need to act for themselves, rather than lobbying the state to act on their behalf.

Consumerism is beginning to have its impact on the health services at both the group and, to a lesser extent, the individual level. At the group level there is a wide range of organizations with different bases, aims and objectives utilising a variety of approaches to achieve their ends.

At the individual level there has been less growth of consumerism in health. It is often difficult for individual patients to be belligerent consumers; they may fear confrontation, or being dismissed as a neurotic or a nuisance. Many fear that in a future emergency requiring professional care, they will be unable to get the help they require. Often individual dissatisfaction is suppressed. The difficulty of battling against a powerful, prestigious and united profession is daunting and it is recognised that such attempts are frequently unsuccessful. However, people with like problems may feel more able to make a firm stand if there is the support of a group.

A NEW PERSPECTIVE?

The changes outlined in this chapter have meant that increasingly both professionals and public have been examining with new interest problems of health and illness and have been looking critically at the services provided.

With the advances in medical technology, there has been at the same time an increased understanding of the need for this to be accompanied by an emphasis on personal care to overcome the real risks of scientific medicine being regarded as cold and inhuman. The varying contribution that different health care professionals can make has been widely discussed and there has been renewed emphasis on the role of the general practitioner in providing continuous and co-ordinated care. (35)

On the other hand with the recognition of the limited contribution of formal medical care in many chronic and behavioural conditions there has been a re-assessment of the contribution that can be made in care and improvement in quality of life by different sections and organizations within the community. With certain groups such as the elderly, the mentally ill and the mentally handicapped there have been policy decisions to change the emphasis from hospital to community care. (36-38) In some places this has meant that there has been a failure to provide sufficient statutory services, particularly when the responsibility has fallen between different statutory bodies. This has in some cases resulted in the burden of care falling on friends and relatives. This enormous burden borne by relatives of the elderly, who are themselves often least equipped to cope, has been demonstrated. (39-40)

The consumer movement has drawn attention to the strengths of community action and protest, and to some of the failings associated with bureaucratic organizations and professional groups. This has encouraged health and health problems to be seen in their community context and not something confined to hospitals or other clinical institutions. The normality of illness has been re-emphasized. The contribution of sociological and anthropological research has done much to remind people of the location and the centrality of health and illness in our society.

In all this there is the discussion of the merits of different approaches, the contribution of individuals and groups and the need to make choices. This includes not only choices between different forms of health care, but choices between health and other demands on government spending such as education, housing, social services or defence. While these may be important policy decisions in the developed countries, they are even more critical in the developing nations where there is poverty, famine, poorly developed services and inadequate manpower. The World Health Organization (41) has called for health care to be made available to everyone by the year 2000, but this requires a new approach to health care and a reassessment of priorities.

Frequently the issues presented by these developments are intensely political. At the two extremes there are demands for a tearing down of the establishment, but these arise from different motives. On the left, women in the more repressive countries have seized power over their own bodies and have instituted their own medical services outside the establishment; here self-help has resulted in collective clinics based on mutual aid. On the right there are demands for de-escalation of formal services, such as the National Health Service on the grounds that the State has encroached far enough on

the freedom of the individual; self-help here means
helping oneself as best one can and letting others
fend for themselves. So the philosophy of
participation in health is claimed by a variety of
ideological sectors which span the political
spectrum.

Mahler (42) has indicated the need to see
'health' rather than 'medicine' as the focus,
although at present there are forces still
encouraging this medical approach in the organized
provision of services.

> The wave of social consciousness in the 19th
> century in Europe and in North America broadened
> our understanding of "Health" but resulted in a
> reaction by the medical Establishment and a
> constriction which is still continuing. By
> legislation, by training, by organization, and
> by the way in which health-related inter-
> ventions are stated and restricted there has
> been a progressive "mystification" in medical
> care which is continuing almost unchecked. As
> our understanding of cause and effect has grown,
> "medicine" has continued to restrict the range
> of problems for which it considers itself
> responsible and the gap between "health care"
> and "medical care" has become even wider. This
> has been coupled with an organisational change
> which has influenced the manner of dealing with
> these problems, a gross restriction in the
> information available and decisions to be made
> by people outside the health professions, and an
> unnecessary but inevitable dependency of the
> population upon the holders of these mysteries.

Mahler looks forward to a 'demystification of
medical technology'. By this he means that choice of
intervention options should be brought nearer to the
consumer, wherever possible. He gives as an example
the treatment of diarrhoeal disease in developing
countries. Rehydration salts for babies should, he
contends, be available to mothers in every home. This
would relieve the mothers of the necessity to attend
special centres for adminstration of the treatment
and take away some of the secrecy of, and thereby
'demystify', a part of medical technology.

Clearly the new perspective is also an old
perspective, but is it a question of retrieving
something that has been lost or building something
new?

NOTES

1.   Elliott-Binns   CP.   An   Analysis   of   Lay
Medicine, Journal of the Royal College of General
Practitioners 1973; 23: 255-264.
2.   Woodward J. and Richards D. Health Care and
Popular   Medicine   in   Nineteenth   Century   England
London: Croom Helm, 1977.
3.   Schofield A. Health at Home Tracts London:
The Religious Tract Society, 1890.
4.   Smiles S. Self-help with Illustrations of
Conduct and Perserverance Centenary edition, London:
John Murray (Publishers) Ltd., 1958.
5.   McKeown   T.   Medicine   in   Modern   Society
London: George Allen and Unwin, 1965.
6.   Wadsworth MEJ. Butterfield WJH. and Blaney
R. Health and Sickness: The   Choice   of   Treatment
London: Tavistock, 1971.
7.   Chadwick   Sir   E.   Report   on   the   Sanitary
Conditions   of   the   Labouring   Population   of   Great
Britain,   1842   Ed.   Flinn   MW.   Edinburgh: Edinburgh
University Press, 1965.
8.   Harris   AI.   Handicapped   and   Impaired   in
Great Britain London: Office of Population Censuses
and Surveys, Social Survey Division, H.M.S.O., 1971.
9.   Sainsbury   S.   Registered   as   Disabled
Occasional   Papers   on   Social   Administration   No 35,
London: The   Social   Administration Research Trust,
1970.
10.   Fry J. Profiles of Disease London: E & S
Livingstone, 1966.
11.   McKeown T. A Historical Appraisal of the
Medical Task. In McLachlan G. & McKeown T.   (Eds.)
Medical History and Medical Care Nuffield Provincial
Hospitals Trust.   London: Oxford University Press,
1971.
12.   Kelman S. The Social Nature of the
Definition Problem in Health. International Journal
of Health Services 1975; 5: 625-641.
13.   Twaddle AC. The Concept of Health Status.
Social Science and Medicine 1974; 8: 29-38.
14.   McHugh   P.   Defining   the   Situation: The
Organisation   of   Meaning   in   Social   Interaction
Indianapolis: The Bobbs-Merrill Co., 1968.
15.   Lemert E. Human Deviance, Social Problems
and   Social   Control   Englewood   Cliffs,   New   Jersey:
Prentice Hall, 1967.
16.   Szasz   TS.   The   Myth   of   Mental   Illness
London: Secker & Warburg, 1962.
17.   Rubington   ES.   and   Weinberg   MS.   (Eds.)
Deviance: The Interactionist Perspective New York:

Macmillan, 1968.
    18. Freidson E. Profession of Medicine - Part
III. The Social Construction of Illness New York:
Dodd Mead & Co., 1970.
    19. Scheff TJ. Being Mentally Ill: A Socio-
logical Theory London: Weidenfeld & Nicholson, 1966.
    20. Selye H. The Stress of Life London:
Longmans, Green & Co., 1956.
    21. Dohrenwend BP. and Dohrenwend BS. (Eds.)
Stressful Life Events: Their Nature and Effects New
York: John Wiley, 1974.
    22. Wolff HS. and Gondell H. Stress and Disease
(2nd edit.) Springfield, Illinois:
C C Thames, 1968.
    23. Levine S. and Scotch NA. (Eds.) Social
Stress Chicago: Aldine Publishing Co., 1970.
    24. Blaxter M. 'Disability' and Rehabilit-
ation: Some Questions of Definition. In Cox C. and
Mead A.   (Eds.) A Sociology of Medical Practice
London: Collier-Macmillan, 1975.
    25. Finlayson A. and McEwen J. Coronary Heart
Disease and Patterns of Living London: Croom Helm,
1977.
    26. Illich I. Medical Nemesis. The Exprop-
riation of Health London: Calder and Boyars, 1974.
    27. Carlson RJ. The End of Medicine New York:
John Wiley, 1975.
    28. Klein R. Who Decides? Pattern of
Authority. British Medical Journal 1978; 2: 73-74.
    29. Powles J. On the Limitations of Modern
Medicine. Science Medicine & Man 1973; 1: 1-34.
    30. Martini CJM. Allan GJB. Davison J. and
Backett EM. Indices Sensitive to Medical Care
Variation. International Journal of Health Services
1977; 7: 293-309.
    31. Gould D. How Doctors Generate Disease. In
Carter CO. and Peel J. (Eds.) Equalities and
Inequalities in Health London: Academic Press, 1976,
105-109.
    32. D'Arcy PF. and Griffin JP. Iatrogenic
Disease London: Oxford University Press, 1979.
    33. Martys CR. Adverse Reactions to Drugs in
General Practice. British Medical Journal 1979; 2:
1194-1197.
    34. Perlman JE. Grassrooting the System.
Social Policy Special Self-Help Issue September/
October 1976; 7,2: 4-20.
    35. Fry J. A New Approach to Medicine.
Priorities and Principles of Health Care Lancaster:
M.T.P. Press, 1978.
    36. Department of Health and Social Security.

A Happier Old Age London H.M.S.O., 1978.
  37. Department of Health and Social Security. Better Services for the Mentally Ill London: H.M.S.O., 1975.
  38. Department of Health and Social Security. Better Services for the Mentally Handicapped London: H.M.S.O., 1971.
  39. Isaacs B., Livingstone M. and Neville Y. Survival of the Unfittest London: Routledge & Kegan Paul, 1972.
  40. Office of Population Census and Surveys. The Elderly at Home London: H.M.S.O., 1978.
  41. Mahler H. Health for all by the Year 2000. WHO Chronicle 1975; 29: 457-461.
  42. Mahler H. Health - A Demystification of Medical Technology. Lancet 1975; 2: 829-833.

Chapter Three

HOW DOES PARTICIPATION ARISE?

In the last chapter we examined some of the factors
that have contributed to the present interest and
commitment to participation.

In the past, individuals had a responsibility
for their own health care usually as a result of
necessity. Families and communities shared their
expertise and their beliefs. Only the relatively
wealthy made use of professional services and the
limited value of such services was well recognized.
As was seen in the last chapter, this gradually
changed with the improved care and intervention
provided by the health services and the free
availability of such care to all. Although there was
widespread participation by the individual in local
health care, there was little participation by the
majority of people in the development of policy
towards health. A few enlightened people, usually
from a position of inherited status, wealth or
academic standing pursued active campaigns to
improve health by a variety of measures. These were
usually accompanied by a wide range of other
humanitarian reforms. When such measures were
applied there was often little direct involvement by
the public, but the public were the beneficiaries of
such activities which resulted in reduced hours of
work, pure water supply, an efficient waste disposal
system and many other reforms.

Today, it appears that there is a different
approach to improving the health and wellbeing of the
population which reflects again the wider aspects of
present social life. There is a demand by individuals
and groups based in the community for active
participation in their own health and for a voice in
the making of policy. At the same time there are
pressures from government which seem to be suggesting
something similar. This chapter will outline the

roles and attitudes of government, professionals and patients, three of the major exponents of the principle of participation.

GOVERNMENT

Why do governments press for participation? Is it expediency, commitment to an ideal, or are motives irrelevant? The dilemmas of government were indicated in the last chapter, but it is necessary to ask what degree of participation in policy-making exists in the National Health Service.

One of the more innovative aspects of government policy in Britain has been the publication of a wide range of discussion and consultative documents. One series, starting with Prevention and Health: Everybody's Business, (1) a reassessment of public and personal health, and then examining specific topics such as pregnancy and childbirth, (2) old age, (3) nutrition, (4) heart disease,(5) alcohol, (6) occupational health (7) was designed for a wide audience, while other publications dealing with priorities (8) and reallocation of resources (9) was aimed at those more directly involved in health service planning and provision. However, many feel that the structure of the National Health Service, from an administrative point of view makes any real participation very limited.

Draper and his colleagues (10) comment that the National Health Service structure resulting from the re-organization of 1974:

> ... restricts the opportunity for co-ordinated and adaptive decision-making, and it certainly reflects a fragmented and mechanistic conception of the objectives of a system of health care delivery. It is in these principal respects that we feel the re-organization has failed ... Furthermore, we believe that such an orientation does not promote participative democracy. Authoritarian bureaucracies aspire to work from the top down: decisions are made at the top of the bureaucracy and, in the bureaucratic ideal, more progressively down to the working level. People at that level are not expected to make the decisions that determine their work nor the conditions under which the work is carried out. When people at the working level are the recipients of services, as in the N.H.S., they are even less expected to

contribute to the processes of deciding what those services should be. The primary obligation of both - providers and recipients is to know their place, and to follow the orders of their betters, that is, the providers, in the case of patients, and hierarchical superiors in the case of providers ... In such systems, people cannot participate in making the decisions which affect them directly.

However, as reported by an editorial in the September 25 1976 issue of BMJ (11)

Richard Crossman promised that the consumer's voice would be represented, and in consequence the community health councils were grafted on to the multi-tier structure late in its embryogenesis, in an attempt to compensate for the lack of democratic election to the health authorities.

In so doing, say Klein and Lewis, (12) "the planners added a gothic folly to the palladian mansion - but in such a way as not to destroy the symmetry (as much intellectual as architectural) of the main building."

By the end of the 1970's consideration was being given to a simplified health service administration, which might be cheaper and less bureaucratic, and by emphasizing the district level of planning might be more sensitive to community needs and responsive to the consumers' point of view. (13) However, almost paradoxically, the abolition of community health councils was suggested in the initial proposals although they were retained when the service reorganized in 1982.

It is interesting to compare the British National Health Service with the service in Quebec which has also undergone reorganization in the last decade. Describing the situation in Canada, Malleson (14) indicates a rather different approach. Claude Castonquay headed a Commission of Inquiry on Health and Social Welfare in the Canadian province of Quebec, which looked into the delivery of health both in Quebec and elsewhere. It found, amongst other things, that Quebec's expensive system was resulting in a very high infant mortality rate and an average life expectancy lower than in other Canadian provinces.

Subsequently, as Minister of Social Affairs, Castonquay put through a Bill whch incorporated the

Commission's findings, emphasizing decentralisation of control and a shift of power to the patients. The basic unit of health care described is a community health centre, providing 80% of health needs, each centre having a board of 10 directors, 5 of whom are elected for a 4 year period by the community.

Studying the Commission's research and the subsequent legislation, Malleson concludes:

> In a world where organizations become bigger and the decisions make procedures more remote and impersonal, such a changeover may keep the problems of health care at a more human and manageable level. By making such a change, we may find that our health services become more efficient and less expensive ...

We do not have the space here to investigate which of these two systems has in practice brought about the greater degree of participation or has lead to an improvement of health, a reduction of illness or improved satisfaction for either professionals or patients. Indeed, as we shall discuss later, few well conducted evaluative studies, to answer such questions, have been carried out.

If participation is introduced in order to achieve a goal however, it surely stands a better chance of being a dynamic force in the system. Whereas, if it is introduced as a token gesture in response to pressure for democratisation, it is unlikely to make an effective contribution to planning and policy making.

The health of the nation's economy is obviously a significant influence on government strategy. Britain has left the boom period of the 1960's and has entered into more sombre times of inflation, cuts in public spending and consciousness of depleted energy sources. This has two implications: one is an urgent investigation into the cost-effectiveness of existing systems; the other is a seeking of 'alternative ways'. Ideas which used to be the prerogative of the social fringes - such as soya beans and solar heat - are now being seriously examined as possible solutions to national problems.

And so those involved in planning and administering the health and social services are looking at the effectiveness and efficiency of the costly National Health Service and wondering whether there might be, somewhere, whole new untapped resources and ideas.

20

PROFESSIONALS

Do professionals want patients to participate more
fully in their health care? The simple answer is that
some do and some don't. Dr John Fry, a general
practitioner, with special interest in self-care,
describes the plight of the conventional doctor,
faced with demands for participation: (15)

> The old and customary view of the physician is
> as a personal physician, friend, philosopher
> and guide through the medical jungle. The
> physician tends to see himself as the leader,
> director, commander, dictator of the medical
> team and services. He feels that he is the
> medical father figure. The medical profession
> seems to have become a gigantic secret society
> which although proclaiming its roles as caring
> for the people's health and diseases, does
> appear to keep its own secrets and to become
> mafia-like at times. It has tended to become
> more inward looking and more concerned with its
> own professional issues and problems than to
> involve itself with social and communal
> problems. In many ways it is a comfortable and
> understandable position for the medical
> profession to hold. It is much easier and less
> stressful to confine work to recognizable
> medical matters within clearly confined bound-
> aries and to avoid moving out.
>   The new ideas of promoting more self-care
> carry with them potential problems and
> difficulties for the physician. They will
> require him to accept a new and less comfortable
> position in medical care. Associated with more
> and better self-care must come more democracy
> and equality for the patient and less power for
> the physician.
>   The patient will have to be treated much
> more as an equal and as a member of the health
> team. The physician will be less of a
> dictatorial self-appointed leader and much more
> as an equal participant in a team. With better
> self-care the physician will have to consider
> what roles the patient can play as an extra
> resource in care. This will create problems in
> defining roles and status and challenges for
> better collaborations and opportunities for
> better organization. The physician will have to
> become a doctor, once more, the teacher,
> philosopher, adviser and guide. He will need to

become much more involved with his local
community in planning, developing and
organizing the local services in a co-
ordinated, rather than in a piecemeal manner.
Such changes will have great implications for
the medical profession, for the universities,
for the community and for the government.

To sell the idea to those who are not so keen,
Fry suggested that doctors will have to be convinced
that it is beneficial not only for the patients, but
also for themselves. This will not be easy. Like
teachers who do not want parents on the school
premises, or nurses who do not want relatives on the
wards, the doctors find it difficult to give up the
idea of an ordered, closed, controllable world and to
believe that if power is taken from them and spread
around in an open-ended and unpredictable
environment, it could result in a better level of
mutual trust and personal fulfillment and a higher
degree of efficiency. They have to learn to have
faith in the patients' ability to be responsible for
themselves before relinquishing their hold; and it is
not a simple matter to implant faith. As indicated
by a symposium published by the British Medical
Journal, some doctors see the answers to problems in
strict demarcation of the contributions by
government, professionals and public, with few areas
of overlap and hence few controversial issues.
(16,17)

My belief is that any society that provides its
citizens with a more-or-less comprehensive
health service can demand a serious return
contribution from them.
This should begin before birth. The
financial allowances given to pregnant women –
maternity leave, grants, etc. – should be
payable only to those who attend early and
regularly for antenatal care. The same
principle – (proved effective by the French)
should be applied to infant health: regular
developmental assessments and attendance at
vaccination clinics should be linked with
financial child benefits. During adult life
insurance companies, building societies, and
other financial institutions could do a lot more
to offer financial incentives to non-smokers
who are not overweight and have their blood
pressure checked regularly.
But the real change in heart needs to come

from the Government. Britain still has a society which is encouraged to see the motor-car as a competitive virility symbol. Motoring needs to be deglamourised - and by so doing cut the accident bill and the numbers of crippled young men. Alcohol, too, needs a new image - as a dangerous and very expensive luxury, not part of the accepted life style. And with a major effort tobacco could be virtually obsolete by the end of the century - especially if its image was linked to old age rather than youth. Too paternalistic? Too much of an infringement of individual freedom? Those who believe in such slogans must explain how they will finance a curative rather than a preventive policy - or introduce a preventive one without sanctions and incentives.

Public participation in health care and preventing disease is steadily increasing and many volunteers are helping the National Health Service. An understanding co-operative public is indeed a great stabilising influence. One further way that the public could help is by reducing their demands on the service. Many illnesses are inevitable, but an appreciable number of physical and mental breakdowns are determined by present-day life styles. The N.H.S. is doing more and more work in hospitals at the foot of the cliff, but what is really needed is a fence at the top, which the public themselves have got to build. Much has been done in simple preventive measures, particularly so far as accidents in the home and elsewhere are concerned, but the next stage is to promote good health by simple measures -brisk daily exercise, maintaining one's weight, developing a preference for unrefined rather than refined cereals, enjoying alcohol only in moderation, smoking less or not at all. Independence, self-reliance, and family stability offer the best protection against the ill-effects of major crises of the body. The N.H.S. will start afresh as soon as it is appreciated that patients must always come first.

Whilst some doctors are blaming patients for their diseases and advocating total acceptance of current medical wisdom as the price of welfare benefits, other doctors are encouraging patients to challenge medical opinion and to participate in their medical care. We see an illustration of this with a recent publication, "How to be your own doctor - sometimes", in which Dr Keith Sehnert (18) creates his new being "the activated patient", who is:

> a kind of hearty hybrid who is three-quarters patient and one-quarter physician. They've learned to speak the doctor's own language, and ask him questions rather than passively sit, honour and obey. They've learned to check vital signs, the first signs of a coronary and how to tell whether a sinus problem is an allergy or a common cold by the colour of the mucous membrane of the nose. They've learned Body Talk - that special language of symptoms that enables them to know what an ache or pain is saying. And they are playing an important and needed role in health partnership with the doctors.

The professional who wants to set up a self-help, independent group could however be faced with certain ethical difficulties. If the group becomes independent, it may take decisions the professional does not like. Such decisions may be of a social or organizational type; for instance, a group may set up a hierarchial structure, reminiscent of the very establishment from which they were hoping to be freed. Or they may be of a medical nature; what if patients decide to act in a way which the doctor knows to be severely detrimental to their health? Professionals must be clear in their own minds whether they are going to allow total freedom or 'freedom' only within limits. The doctor who has started out with the aim of reducing the workload by encouraging patients to self-treat "trivial" illness may find that there is an increased demand from more sophisticated and educated patients seeking reassurance for their self-treatment, that patients present with more complex problems in place of the "trivial" or that consultations do not take place until the "trivial" problems have become serious.

So, patient participation is an issue which doctors will have to face. There are those who have yet to come to terms with the idea. And for those who already have, there are multi-faceted problems to work on; the doctor-patient relationship of generations is not going to be easily replaced; a new formula has to be found.

It is perhaps not surprising that Claflin describes the situation as follows:

> There is no small irony when one views the self-

help movement and sees a primary impediment to
its maximum potential effectiveness being the
very individuals, with the highest levels of
education in the community, who describe
themselves as 'care givers' or as having
membership in the 'helping professions'. (19)

PATIENTS

For patients wishing to participate in their own
health, there are various possible relationships
with the professionals. The discussion here will
primarily consider the role of patient groups,
although most of the points are also applicable to
the individual patient. In considering these,
though, it is necessary first to recognise the
inevitable dependence of the population on its
doctors and nurses.

One cause of this is their expertise, which
means that when a statement is made, patients cannot
tell whether it is an unchallengeable statement of
scientific fact or prejudice or self-interested
opinions, masquerading as fact. And when it is
patients' own health, possibly their lives, which are
at stake, it never seems to be the right time to
challenge.

Increased self-care for haemophiliacs in the
United States of America has given rise to anxiety
amongst professionals about consequential decrease
in doctor-patient visits. At a recent conference,
Segal (20) commented that it was question-nable
whether such concern was genuine or merely a
maneouvre for professional and institutional
maintenance.

The second cause of groups' dependence is the
adminstrative monopoly of the medical establishment
over illness. Only professionals have the power to
legitimate illness and therefore groups which are
often dependent on doctors referring patients to
them, fear that such referrals will only be made to
approved groups. Groups then have to decide upon the
type of relationship they aim to achieve with the
health professionals, weighing up their need to be
'approved' with the task of offering real
alternatives.

Co-operation
Some groups work in close co-operation with doctors.
Such groups have many patients referred by doctors;

their conferences are attended by specialists who also help prepare their pamphlets. This close co-operation has the advantages of exchanging knowledge and breaking down barriers. But it can also have the disadvantage of subordination to professionals and to their ideology. Instead of fellow sufferers, bonded by common difficulties, exchanging problems and comfort, it could lead to the members becoming, in Dewar's (21) words "professionalised clients", that is patients who see through the professional's eyes and speak the professional's language. Because the "professionalised client" is more interested in applying the professional treatment, than in what is effective, he or she serves only to reinforce the feelings among other members of impotence and isolation that come with being a client.

Conflict and Separation

For other groups the keynote is conflict or separatism. This is more evident in other countries, such as Italy, where conflict is perhaps more readily provoked because of the greater rigidity of the medical system. This is not to say, however, that Great Britain is immune from such challenges. There are advantages to the situation when development of such movements is separated from professional or formal organization. Many express the hope that an anti-system bias should limit bureaucratisation and some of the negative consequences of institutional-isation. Levin and his colleagues (22) comment on the possibility that professionals will seek to dominate self-care initiatives, thus compromising their viability.

The new perspective demands that self-help groups should not have to fit into the existing framework, built around professionals, but that professionals should have to fit in with people. The growth of participation should not be seen as a new sort of health-care, with a concomitant burgeoning of professionalism and expertise but as a move back to first principles, an effort to remove the blinkers that professionalism has imposed upon individuals, a dismantling of the structure whereby others have come to have more power over individuals than they have themselves.

It must be noted however, that there could be disadvantages for those groups in conflict with the professionals, namely that its subversive activity could cut people off from the benefits offered by mainstream medical technology. This dilemma will be seen to have been tackled by the Women's Movement which has attempted to accept some of the medical technology, but reject the method of handing it out.

SELF-HELP GROUPS AND NATIONAL HEALTH SERVICES

"When the counter-culture develops something of value, the establishment rips it off and sells it back." (23) Cartner and Riessman have proposed that self-help groups be the key to planning for management of chronic diseases. (24) To assess whether this is realistic, it is necessary to remember the distinction between those groups in conflict, and those working in co-operation, with the professionals.

Many groups - both professionally, and lay, inspired - are already closely associated with the National Health Service - for instance, self-help mastectomy groups based in hospitals. It is, however, difficult to plan self-help groups, because self-help groups are essentially voluntary. 'Planning' and 'policies' are not appropriate terms. All that can be said, in a policy-making way, is the groups have official approval and that funds are available.

Many groups such as The Patients Association and the Disabled Income Group, seek specifically to influence policy and service provision. As for those groups 'beyond the pale', it may well happen that their methods will be copied by establishment groups and that their function will be recognised as worthwhile and included in the state service, but it is in this way that breakaway groups have become part of the evolution of the State Health services.

It is unlikely that the need for, or the contribution of independent groups will be ruled out in the foreseeable future.

SOME RESERVATIONS

The risks involved in participation are examined in relevant chapters but there are some objections in principle to participation which might profitably be stated:
1. Self-care must not be a euphemism for cost-cutting particularly at a time of widespread economic constraints. Criticism of the over-medicalisation of people's lives or problems must not mask the undoubted gaps in the health service. The Black Report (25) documents clearly the continuing and indeed worsening inequalities in health in Britain

between the different socio-economic groups. There is a certain lunacy about treatment being denied to those who want and need it (the thousands who are waiting for hospital beds, the need for continuing care units, the desperate shortage of short-term care to relieve overburdened families of handicapped children or senile parents) and yet forced on those who do not want it and possibly may not need it, or allowed to those who want but don't need it (the placebo prescription). Similarly there is a need to examine the problems of inappropriate care and the varying contributions of the different caring professions. Certainly self-care may be called for in some areas, but more professional care may be needed in others.

2. A second criticism is that self-help addresses itself to the symptoms of the problem rather than causes. Rather than providing what is not provided by the State, it could be said that groups should pressure the State into allotting them a fair share of the resources. In reply to this, it is argued that:

(a) grouping together can raise consciousness about the shortcomings of the State and result in people becoming more politically active.

(b) this introduces the tricky question of where the obligations of the Welfare State stop. Should the State be made to provide all our health care? Or is there an inherent value in groups being outside the establishment?

3. The third reservation is perhaps the most subtle and the most difficult to resolve. The proliferation of self-help groups is an indication that people do not just 'live' any more, they 'cope'. In debates about why self-help groups are so middle-class, it is suggested that working class people have their own 'coping networks' (otherwise known as families). (26,27) This is connected with the view that life should be happy, so sadness is interpreted as depression, an aberration requiring treatment. Life should be smooth, so when people meet obstacles, they need a coping mechanism - in some cases a self-help group.

Perhaps this is over-sceptical; perhaps the coping approach is a sound response to the nature of modern society, and more particularly, to the nature of middle class culture where 'coping in groups' is most apparent, a break-out from the stiff upper lip and the tight nuclear family.

But it is as well to bear in mind the hypothesis that sometimes 'coping' and self-help groups might be a professional approach to what is in fact, just living.

PROFESSIONALS AND THE SELF-HELP MOVEMENT

The relationship between professionals and self-help groups is a key question. Movement towards participation has to be a two-way process: the doctors giving, and the patients taking, power and responsibility.

Among doctors, there is immense diversity of opinion. Some favour the traditional paternalistic doctor/patient relationship and some press for a radical shift of power from the doctor to the patient. Tradition, training, prejudices and rituals are important in any professional group. (28,29)

As for the patients, there are many who do not want to accept responsibility for their own health and treatment. Among those who do, some enter into participation gradually with the permission of the professionals and others seize power unilaterally. Their relationships with the professionals can be co-operative or conflicting; both have benefits and risks. (30)

These relationships and other aspects of participation will be discussed further in subsequent chapters, but it must be registered at this stage, that how professionals act and react towards patient participation is a major issue.

EVALUATION

There is a consciousness that conventional methods of evaluation are not applicable in looking at the effectiveness of self-help groups; their worth cannot properly be assessed in simple statistics of traditional indicators of morbidity and mortality, and some writers distinguish between 'hard' and 'soft' evidence. There are the individual success stories, measurable in the facts and figures of organizations such as Weight Watchers and Alcoholics Anonymous and there are the less easily measurable factors such as satisfaction expressed by members, the flourishing nature of the groups and, on a theoretical level, properties which are, in principle, more likely to be health-giving than the traditional role of the passive patient. Few studies have been comparative or have considered 'outcome measures'.

A useful distinction can be made, also, between the 'personal' and 'technical' services offered by groups. It would seem that personal needs, such as for emotional support, might be better met by mutual groups than by doctors, but this is difficult to quantify and compare. As for technical services, such as exercises or dietary advice, there are standards of objective evaluation which can be applied.

Some of those who participate in self-help groups would argue that evaluation is neither necessary nor appropriate, that it is self-evident that they help people with problems who have not been helped by formal services. With the increasing contribution of the social and behavioural sciences in health services research, which has resulted in new tools, better able to evaluate quality of care and quantity of life, it would seem that there is now an opportunity to examine carefully and sympathetically, the various contributions made by different organizations and different approaches.

NOTES

1. Department of Health and Social Security. Prevention and Health: Everybody's Business London: H.M.S.O., 1977.

2. Department of Health and Social Security. Reducing the Risk London: H.M.S.O., 1977.

3. Department of Health and Social Security. A Happier Old Age London: H.M.S.O., 1978.

4. Department of Health and Social Security. Eating for Health London: H.M.S.O., 1978.

5. Department of Health and Social Security. Avoiding Heart Attacks London: H.M.S.O., 1981.

6. Department of Health and Social Security. Drinking Sensibly London: H.M.S.O., 1981.

7. Health and Safety Commission. Occupational Health Services: The Way Ahead London: H.M.S.O., 1977.

8. Department of Health and Social Security. The Way Forward: Priorities in the Health and Social Services London: H.M.S.O., 1977.

9. Department of Health and Social Security. Sharing Resources for Health in England London: H.M.S.O., 1976.

10. Draper P., Grenholm G. and Best G. The Organization of Health Care: A Critical View of the 1974 Reorganization of the National Health Service. In Tuckett D. (Ed.) An Introduction to Medical Sociology London: Tavistock, 1976.

11. Editorial. What Does the Community Care

About. British Medical Journal 1976; 2: 720.

12. Klein R. and Lewis J. The Politics of Consumer Representation London: Centre for Studies in Social Policy, 1976.

13. Department of Health and Social Security. Patients First. Consultative Paper on the Structure and Management of the National Health Service in England and Wales London: H.M.S.O., 1979.

14. Malleson A. Need Your Doctor be so Useless? London: George Allen & Unwin, 1973.

15. Fry J. Self-Care. Role of the Patient in Primary Health Care. The Viewpoint of the Medical Practitioner Paper submitted at the symposium on the Role of the Individual in Primary Health Care. Copenhagen, Denmark: 11-15 August 1973.

16. Smith T. Prevention or Cure. British Medical Journal 1978; 2: 24.

17. Avery Jones Sir F. Getting the National Health Service Back on Course. British Medical Journal 1978; 2: 5-9.

18. Sehnert KW. How to be your Own Doctor - Sometimes New York: Grossett and Dunlap, 1975.

19. Claflin B. Alcoholics Anonymous: One Million Members and Growing. In Self Help and Health: A Report New Human Services Institute, Queens College, C.U.N.Y., 1976, 57-62.

20. Segal B. Quoted in Briggs HC. Conference on Self Help and Health: Summary of Discussion. In Self Help and Health: A Report Opus Cit. p.4.

21. Dewar T. Professionalized Clients as Self Helpers. In Self Help and Health: A Report Opus Cit. 77-83.

22. Levin LS., Katz AH. and Holst E. Self Care. Lay Initiatives in Health London: Croom Helm, 1977.

23. Geiger J. Quoted in Jencks SF. Problems in Participatory Health Care. In Self Help and Health: A Report Opus Cit. 85-98.

24. Gartner A. and Riessman F. Self Help Models and Consumer-Intensive Health Practice. American Journal of Public Health 1976; 66: 783-786.

25. Department of Health and Social Services. Inequalities in Health Report of a Research Working Group (Black). London: D.H.S.S., 1980.

26. Bott E. Family and Social Network. Roles, Norms and External Relationships in Ordinary Urban Families London: Tavistock, 1971.

27. McKinlay J. Social Networks and Utilization Behaviour. Social Forces 1973; 5: 1: 275-294.

28. Freidson E. Professional Dominance: The Social Structure of Medical Care New York: Atherton Press, 1970.

29. Bloom SW. <u>The Doctor and His Patient</u> New York: The Free Press, 1965.

30. Bloor MJ. and Horobin GW. Conflict and Conflict Resolution. In Doctor/Patient Interaction. In Cox C. and Mead A. (Eds.) <u>A Sociology of Medical Practice</u> London: Collier-Macmillan, 1973. 285-298.

Chapter Four

HEALTH AND ILLNESS: THE SOCIAL SETTING

Health and illness occur in a social setting and cannot be considered in isolation from the traditions, culture, values and structure of a society, or from an individual's or society's chosen way of coping with problematic issues. (1,2)

Starting with the pioneer work of the Peckham Health Centre, (3) community studies (4,5,6) have clearly shown how normal it is for individuals to experience symptoms, and the varying ways in which these are defined determine the action taken. (7,8) Only a proportion of those symptoms are even discussed within the family context and fewer still are mentioned to those outside the family - friends and colleagues at work. They may be discussed with someone with experience - possibly in the health field or perhaps the foreman at work, just because he is the person who normally gives advice. Only a small proportion of the original symptoms will be brought formally to the health professionals. This has been described as the 'iceberg' of disease. (9,10)

PATHWAYS TO CARE

Illness usually presents initially in a family context (11-13) and it is often forgotten by professionals that the first assessment of symptoms and frequently the first diagnosis is made by the individual with the symptom, sometimes assisted by a member of the family or a friend. When consultation with a professional occurs, it may be for reassurance on either the diagnosis or the action taken, as well as for professional diagnosis and prescription. (14,15) Depending on an individual's social or occupational situation, formal legitimation of illness may be required to enable the patient to receive the state benefits linked to sickness absence from work.

This discussion of health issues, particularly of symptoms, through a lay hierarchy of experts, or the 'lay referral system' (16) as it has been termed, and the use of 'lay consultants' is well documented. Its exact nature varies according to the culture and social networks that exist in particular communities. (17,18,19) It is interesting to note that the system not only operates prior to consultation with a doctor but the advice and treatment dispensed is equally discussed back through the lay referral system and if the professional advice is incongruent with the local culture it may be rejected.

In the process of defining the situation, amongst other things, individuals use their 'stock of knowledge' which as Schutz (20,21) and McHugh (22) point out is an accumulation of their own direct experience, their knowledge of others' experience, the influence of the media and thus it represents the results of the continuing process of socialization. The 'stocks of knowledge' of the lay person and the professional will be different. Interaction may lead to a shared definition of the problem or the definitions may remain incongruous. (23-28) The relative power of the parties involved in the interaction must be taken into account. (29,30) The very word 'patient', the one who suffers, describes one who submits to the authority of the skilled professional who knows what is best.

It is probable that this process of definition is not radically different from other social situations where definitions of 'normality and abnormality' are discussed. How is normality defined? Who is responsible for the definition - the patient, the family, the doctor or society? If the doctor defines departure from normality as a biological (pathological) measure and the patient is concerned with function or behaviour there may be problems in reaching a shared definition. Drawing together some existing theoretical approaches it is possible to outline a simple model of the process of seeking care. (31,32,33)

In a problematic situation, after the process of definition, the choice of action is made from a set of possible lines of response. (20,21,34) Just as the individual's definition is the product of his or her life history, of experience, both social and individual, both direct and vicarious, through connection with others, so is his or her choice of 'recipes for action'. If a symptom is defined as a trivial departure from normal it may be ignored and left to vanish of its own accord. If defined as trivial but recognized as a common minor ailment, appropriate home remedies may be applied, or widely advertised modern cures may be purchased from the chemist or supermarket. If there is a more serious symptom which is thought to be related to major illness, there may be rapid recourse to a medical practitioner. The individual with symptoms, based on a previous experience, begins by prescribing delay, in the knowledge that most symptoms go away (the majority of illnesses are self-limiting). Later, if the symptoms persist, self-treatment is instituted usually with tried and personally tested remedies that produce symptomatic relief. This may be encouraged by previous contact with professionals who had prescribed similar symptomatic treatments for similar symptoms. Only at a later stage, if symptoms persist beyond the normal limit, become worse, interfere with everyday activities or in some way are recognized as potentially threatening, is there an approach to professionals for diagnosis and treatment. This is often the result of the advice to seek such care from those consulted in the lay referral system. (35,36)

To some, illness is seen as a normal trivial matter which should be dealt with by the quickest and most expedient resources available. To others, illness speaks of possible death - any departure from the individual's norm is taken as an indication of human frailty and reminds people that they are mortal. (37,38,39) Many factors such as the social system, particularly social class and social networks and the general cultural and religious beliefs, as well as the severity or chronicity of symptoms are likely to affect the presentation of symptoms to medical care. (18,19,40-45) In some groups and individuals, interference with function is more important than pain or feelings, while in others, pain may be regarded as more significant. (46) Much depends on the way that health and illness are defined.

SOME DEFINITIONS OF HEALTH

Oxford Dictionary (47)   - Soundness of body: that condition in which its function is duly discharged.

W.H.O. (48)	- A state of complete physical, mental and social well being.
Parsons (49)	- Health may be defined as the state of optimum capacity of an individual for the effective perfor-mance of valued tasks.
Rossdale (50)	- The product of a harmonized relationship between man and his ecology.
Dubos (51)	- A modus vivendi enabling imperfect men to achieve a rewarding and not too painful existence while they cope with an imper-fect world.

These few definitions illustrate the differences in approach - some emphasizing an ideal state -
some concentrating on a practical approach. Some are
more concerned with physical conditions - others are
based on a broader perspective, involving feelings,
relationships or functions. Is health to be seen in
absolute terms, or, as Wilson (52) does, as
situational?

> that is, related to what people believe to be
> the fullness of life for them. It is an
> expression of qualities to which they give
> value, and because they must choose between
> different factors in a world of limited
> resources, ethico-political decisions are
> involved. Health is estimated by many criteria
> drawn from every corner of a people's life,
> including their capacity for enriching
> interpersonal relationships.

Is health a right? Is illness abnormal? What is
the relationship between illness and other problems
and suffering? Herzlich (53) notes that:

> anthropologists and historians of medicine are
> in general agreement that causal conceptions of
> illness - whether popular notions or medical
> theories - range between two extremes. On the
> one hand, illness is indigenous to man, and the
> individual carries it in embryo; the ideas of
> resistance to disease, heredity and predispos-
> ition are here the key concepts. On the other
> hand, illness is thought of as exogenous; man is

naturally healthy and illness is due to the action of an evil will, a demon or sorcerer, noxious elements, emanations from the earth or microbes, for example.

She suggests that the individual would appear to feel himself responsible for his health, because good or bad it defines him and suggests the hypothesis that the individual may feel guilty for having allowed his health to be impaired, rather than for having caught the actual disease. He feels guilty for having lost his health. Sickness and suffering may be seen by different religions as punishment for individual sin, punishment for the sin of mankind (or just the inevitable consequence of this), a result of insufficient faith or trust in a god, or alternatively something that is of value, purposefully permitted by their god, which would lead to a better quality of life.

HEALTH AND ILLNESS BEHAVIOUR

As already noted, health is a social value, (1,2,40,41, 54,55) and it must be seen alongside other values. The behaviour of individuals as groups is related to the culture, the existing services and many other social variables. Health may be sacrificed to ambition or expediency or for the good of others. Discussion of definitions of health and illness is not an academic matter with no practical implications, but the beliefs and the attitudes of patients, family, friends, professionals of differing kinds and society (or sub-groups in society) influence the diagnosis of illness, the action taken, the services offered, the utilization of these services, the treatment (or in some cases the punishment) prescribed and the outcome. (45,56,57,58,59)

The changing attitudes and therefore the appropriate treatments for what is currently called mental illness is an excellent example - demon possession, witchcraft, madness, mental illness, problems of living - the labels are different and the treatments are different, as are the social attitudes. There are different definitions by law and medicine. The intervention of a psychiatrist may lead to a different label, detention in a different institution and a longer or indeterminate sentence of separation from the community. (60,61)

What definitions, for example are attached to alcoholism, (when does alcohol intake become

excessive?) sexual deviations or variations, hypo-
chondriasis and malingering by individuals with
different backgrounds and experience in the various
cultural groups within present day society? Custom,
fashion and fad are all important. The health
behaviour of last century or the 1920's would hardly
be recongized today. While many sympathise with
Shaw's (62) view of the medical profession, as a
conspiracy against the laity, the seeking of 'septic
foci' is no longer so fashionable. Today in
industrialised society it is accepted as normal that
30% of the population have backache and that large
numbers of people are killed on the roads each year.
Different problems are seen as normal in developing
countries, where infectious disease, parasites,
civil war, poverty and malnutrition are common.
    The contribution of the social and psycholog-
ical sciences has done much to broaden the
understanding of health and illness. (63-67) In
addition to considering the pathological, psychological or bacteriological aspects of disease, the
significance of the condition for the individual and
those associated, the impact of illness on society
and the complex inter-relationship of social factors
has led to a more holistic approach. Health and
illness in the societal aspects have become an object
of study and a proper concern of health
professionals. (68,69) Similarly with the development of interest in environment and ecology, there
has been a renewal of interest in the influence of
physical as well as social factors on health. (52)
This is currently illustrated by the increasing
discussion of the issues associated with life in the
inner city areas (70-72) and the close relationship
between health, housing, leisure, life style, life
events and life chances. (73-77) One particular area
where there have been specific developments is the
field of health and work. (78)

RESPONSIBLITY FOR HEALTH

Normally people are not blamed for being ill - even
if they are suffering from sports injuries. There
are however ambivalent attitudes to those presenting
with conditions such as suicidal attempts and
venereal disease. Certain conditions and the
consequences of certain acts have 'moral' overtones
for both individuals and society. Discussions of the
value and limitations of Parsons's (79-81) 'Sick
Role' has been one of the mainstays of medical

sociology for over twenty years. Patients are not considered responsible for their condition and are exempted from normal social roles and responsibilities. It is considered necessary for them to be aided in their recovery, but they are to co-operate with those who provide the expert help and advice. Similarly, the question of labelling and legitimation have been thorny issues and these have been related to the debate as to whether or not illness can be examined in the wider context of social deviance, thus providing an alternative way of examining health and illness instead of the traditional medical model. (16,61,82,83)

Illich (84) has drawn attention to the medicalisation of problems, and his writings have stimulated much discussion and continuing controversy. Given the highly visible miracles of medicine, there has been a tendency for difficult problems either to be pushed towards the medical profession or for the profession to seek to extend its already considerable sphere of activity. Sometimes the fact that the technology is medically based, eg. family planning and abortion, has encouraged a medical assumption of the wider field.

In Illich's view:

> Health has ceased to be a native endowment each man is presumed to possess until proven ill, and has become the ever-distant promise to which one is entitled by virtue of social justice ...

> In a morbid society the environment is so rearranged that for most of the time most people lose their power and will for self-sufficiency and finally cease to believe that autonomous action is feasible ... The result is a morbid society that demands universal medicalisation and a medical establishment that certifies universal morbidity.

> In a morbid society the belief prevails that defined and diagnosed ill health is infinitely preferrable to any other form of negative label. It is better than criminal or political deviance, better than laziness, better than self-chosen absence from work. More and more people subconsciously know that they are sick and tired of their jobs and of their leisure passivities, but they want to be lied to and told that physical illness relieves them of social and political responsiblities. They want their doctor to act as lawyer and priest. As a lawyer, the doctor exempts the patient from his

normal duties and enables him to cash in on the insurance fund he was forced to build. As a priest the doctor becomes an accomplice for the patient creating the myth that he is an innocent victim of biological mechanisms rather than a lazy, greedy or envious deserter of a social struggle for control over the tools of production. Social life becomes a give and take of therapy, medical, psychiatric, pedagogic or genetic.

Kosa and Zola (85) show how the day to day routines become of prime importance:

> The practising physician, a proverbially busy person, tends to regard health, illness, disability and death in their concrete relevance. For him, the problem is how to diagnose the specific complaints presented by the patient and how to apply the treatment that is appropriate under the given circumstances. His attention centres around such practical details as the heart murmur of a middle aged man, the examination of a healthy child, or the emotional difficulties of a suburban housewife. Amid such preoccupations, definitions of health and illness appear to him as matters all too abstract and removed from the current problems

- yet he is using definitions, he is constrained by his theories of illness and the concepts he has of his patients.

Illich (86) sums up his view of health, and clearly indicates that it is not something which can be treated as a separate entity, but is an integral part of daily life.

> Health designates a process of adaption. It is not the result of instinct, but of an autonomous yet culturally shaped reaction to socially created reality. It designates the ability to adapt to changing environments, to growing up and to ageing, to healing when damaged, to suffering and to the peaceful expectation of death. Health embraces the future as well, and therefore includes anguish and the inner resources to live with it.

In one sense, it is clearly ridiculous to think that an individual is not participating in his or her own health. Daily the individual in his or her social setting makes decisions about health promoting activities, avoidance of situations and activities which may endanger health or appear unsafe. At the first sign of illness, the individual draws on personal experience, consults others and makes decisions about self care, a visit to the doctor, or alternative sources of help or advice. It is principally when in contact with the health professions that least participation appears to take place, although in the recovery phase, especially if there is prolonged rehabilitation, individuals may reassume much of the responsiblity for their own care. During the whole process, from health, through illness to recovery, the patient may experience a number of different 'roles' with varying amounts of participation.

A framework which has been found useful to aid in the understanding of this process of redefinition and making of choices in a chronological sequence is the concept of 'career'. In recent years this has been extended from its occupational origin to other areas of behaviour such as that of mental patients by Goffman, (87) tuberculosis patients by Roth, (88) and parents of polio patients by Davis. (89) This not only encourages health and illness to be seen in a longitudinal manner where episodes are not considered as isolated entities but enables comparison of possible different pathways related to different service provision or differing choice between these services. Lemert (90) considers that this process should not be seen as fixed stages which patients must pass through but it refers to recurrent or typical contingencies and problems awaiting patients according to the particular type of career patterns, with the added notion that there may be theoretically 'best' choices set into a situation by presenting technology and social structure. This clearly sets individual participation in the social context including the formal health services with the final outcome being the result of the interaction between the many participants. Szasz and Hollander (91) have described three models of doctor-patient interaction which occur during the process of illness. Initially there is the phase of Activity-Passivity - where the physician 'actually does something to the patient' who only acts as a 'passive recipient'. There is the second phase of Guidance-Co-operation, where the physician 'tells the patient what to do and the patient acts as co-operator'. Finally, there is the Mutual Co-operation phase, during which the physician 'helps the patient to help himself' and the patient acts as an active participant in the partnership. Frequently, both patients and doctors may find difficulty in accepting these roles and often in the practical situation, the issues are much less clear.

Thus the debate as to the factors responsible for ill health continues, with no clear separation between factors related directly to the individual's physical body, social circumstances and personal behaviour and the wider physical, economic, industrial and social environment. Attempts are made to determine the environmental determinants of cancer (92) or to clarify the contribution of life events or other social causes. (93,94)

This has an added significance because of the influence that such studies have on policy. Who is responsible for promoting health and preventing disease? What is to be the contribution of the individual and what is to be the contribution of authorities? What problems can be seen in terms of individual action and for what problems is it inappropriate to suggest individual action?

Currently with the economic problems that exist in many countries, there is a desire for cheaper solutions, there is discussion of priorities, of choosing between alternative paths of action and of limitations in budgets. (95-97) In the desire for a new approach, there is often an emphasis on the increased role of the individual in solving problems, although this is less common in official government reports, but is there a risk of misuse? Illich has clearly called for a re-emphasis on the individual role in health. However, as Navarro (98) points out the solution to social problems cannot be seen solely in terms of the individual. Citing three current major health problems, alienation of the individual in society, occupational diseases and cancer, he argues that:

> These are just three examples of the economic and political aetiology of disease, and this aspect is as apparent today as when our diseases were predominantly infectious ones. But, and as one would expect, the response of the powerful in society is either to deny or obscure that reality. Instead, the cause of the problem is perceived as individual, and the nature of intervention is individually oriented (health education in prevention and clinical medicine in cure). Consequently, one of today's most active state policies at the central government

level in most Western capitalist countries is to
encourage and stimulate these health programmes, such as health education, that are aimed at
bringing about changes in the individual but not
in the economic or political environment.

It is interesting to note that while much
of the disease affecting the working class in
Engel's time was supposedly due to the poor
moral fibre of the workmen and their families,
today the poor health conditions of that class
and the majority of the population are assumed
to be due to their lack of concern for their own
health and their poor health education. In both
cases, the solution to our public lack of health
is   individual   prevention   and   individual
therapy.

It is all too easy for authorities to seek to
blame individuals and to transfer to individuals the
responsibility for collective failures. Illich (99)
considers that "the level of public health
corresponds to the degree to which the means and
responsibility for coping with illness are
distributed amongst the total population."
Navarro (100) goes further:

I would encourage you to think of social
medicine and public health not only in terms of
improving water and sewage systems, or even in
terms of improving occupational medicine, but
also and previously (as did the founders of
social medicine) in terms of redistributing the
economic and political power in our society from
a few to the many. Indeed, Virchow, the founder
of social medicine, clearly saw the need to
merge the medical task with the political and
social forces. Medicine is a social science and
politics is medicine on a large scale.

He goes on to say that:

In summary, I perceive the public health task as
serving and supporting the public's demands not
only for health resources, but also for control
of them and all the resources they produce. But
in order to undertake that task, it is necessary
to realize that we cannot have a progressive
health movement in the absence of a progressive
political movement.

A slightly different perspective has been put

forward by Mahler (101) who has been responsible for a considerable change in emphasis within the World Health Organization.

> What I am advocating, for industrial as well as the developing world, is for the health establishment to make a major effort to describe all the health problems and the alternating ways of dealing with them in an objective way and to accept a national decision making process based on the evidence.

As Pill and Stott (102) point out, in the debate on individual responsibility

> what is missing, however, both in the official documents and the criticisms of them, is any discussion of how members of the general public may feel about the onus for illness being shifted on to the individual. The establishment of just what the concept of individual responsibility for health means to various groups in our society would seem to be a necessary first step in assessing how effective official policy on preventive health is likely to be and formulating appropriate strategies for behaviour change.

From their study of a sample of working class mothers they concluded that at least half held fatalistic views about illness causation and were prepared to accept the concept of blame only under very restricted circumstances involving direct risk taking.

The authors suggest three possible hypotheses which are not necessarily mutually exclusive and which arise from their demonstration that an important sector of society appears to be resistant to the adoption of feelings of responsiblity for health as promoted by official bodies through traditional health education techniques.

1.   That a sector of society is immutably resistant to change and so fixed in their ways that personal changes are unlikley to be achieved.
2.   That innovation in health education and prevention can still achieve better results with the 'resistant' sector of society.
3.   That a large sector of society is trapped in socio-economic circumstances which render the officially recommended choices of lifestyle either impractical or irrelevant, however much the

individuals may desire to change.

Despite the gravity of these hypotheses Pill and Stott end their article on a hopeful note "Extensive opportunities for innovation in both operational studies and fundamental research now lie before those who are prepared to try to bury their biases and embark on the tempting yet trying process of interdisciplinary work in health promotion".

NOTES

1. Herzlich C. Health and Illness. A Social Psychological Analysis Translated by Graham D. European Monographs in Social Psychology London: Academic Press, 1973.

2. Dubos R. Man Adapting New Haven: Yale University Press, 1965.

3. Pearse IH. The Quality of Life. The Peckham Approach to Human Ethology Edinburgh: Scottish Academic Press, 1979.

4. Wadsworth MEJ., Butterfield WJH. and Blaney R. Health and Sickness: The Choice of Treatment London: Tavistock, 1971.

5. Fry J. Profiles of Disease. A Study of the Natural History of Common Diseases Edinburgh: E & S Livingstone, 1966.

6. Horder J. and Horder E. Illness in General Practice. Practitioner 1954; 173: 177-87.

7. Field D. The Social Definition of Illness. In Tuckett D. (Ed.) An Introduction to Medical Sociology London: Tavistock, 1976, 334-366.

8. Kelman S. The Social Nature of the Definition Problem in Health. International Journal of Health Services 1975; 5: 625-641.

9. Morris JN. Uses of Epidemiology 3rd edition. Edinburgh: Churchill Livingstone, 1975. Chapter 6.

10. Hannay DR. The Symptom Iceberg - A Study of Community Health London: Routledge and Kegan Paul, 1979.

11. Chen E. and Cobb S. Family Structure in Relation to Health and Disease. Journal of Chronic Diseases 1960; 12: 544-567.

12. Special Issue. Family, health and illness. Journal of Comparative Family Studies 1973; 4.

13. Hansen DA. and Hill R. Families under Stress. In: Christensen HT. (Ed.) Handbook of Marriage and the Family Chicago: Rand McNally, 1964.

14. Bell J., Black IJ., McEwen J. and Pearson JCG. Patterns of Illness and Use of Services in a New Town: A Preliminary Report. Public Health

1979; 93: 333-343.

15. Stimson GV. and Webb B. Going to see the Doctor: The Consultation Process in General Practice London: Routledge and Kegan Paul, 1975.

16. Freidson E. Profession of Medicine New York: Dodds Mead & Co., 1970.

17. Bott E. Family and Social Network 2nd edition. London: Tavistock, 1971.

18. Finlayson A. Social Networks as Coping Resources, Lay Help and Consultation Patterns used by Women in Husbands Post Infarction Careers. Social Science and Medicine 1976; 10: 97-10.

19. McKinlay J. Social Networks and Utilization Behaviour. Social Forces 1973; 51: 275-292.

20. Schutz A. Collected papers. The Problems of Social Reality Natanson M. (Ed.) The Hague: Martinus Nijhoff, 1962.

21. Schutz A. The Stranger. In Collected Papers II Studies in Social Theory. Brodersen A. (Ed.) The Hague: Martinus Nijhoff, 1964.

22. McHugh P. Defining the Situation. The Organisation of Meaning in Social Interaction Indianapolis: Bobbs Merrill, 1968.

23. Tuckett D. Doctors and Patients. In Tuckett D. (Ed.) An Introduction to Medical Sociology London: Tavistock, 1976. Chapter 6.

24. Cartwright A. Human Relations and Hospital Care Lordon: Routledge and Kegan Paul, 1964.

25. Cartwright A. Patients and their Doctors London: Routledge and Kegan Paul, 1967.

26. Freidson E. Patients views of Medical Practice New York: Russell Sage Foundation, 1962.

27. Zola IK. Problems of Communication, Diagnosis and Patient Care. Journal of Medical Education 1963; 28: 829-838.

28. Thomas WS. and Thomas DS. The Child in America New York: Knopf, 1928.

29. Blau PM. Exchange and Power in Social Life New York: John Wiley, 1964.

30. Homans G. Social Behaviour: Its Elementary Forms London: Routledge and Kegan Paul, 1961.

31. Rosenstock IM. What Research on Motivation Suggests for Public Health. American Journal of Public Health 1960; 50: 295-302.

32. Suchman EA. Stages of Illness and Medical Care. Journal of Health and Human Behaviour 1965; 6: 114-128.

33. Mechanic D. Medical Sociology. A Selective View New York: The Free Press, 1968. Chapter 4.

34. Rose AM. A Systematic Summary of Symbolic Interaction Theory. In Rose AM. (Ed.) Human Behaviour

and Social Process London: Routledge and Kegan Paul, 1962. Chapter 1.

35. Tuckett D. Becoming a Patient. In Tuckett D. (Ed.) An Introduction to Medical Sociology London: Tavistock, 1976. Chapter 5.

36. Robinson D. The Process of Becoming Ill London: Routledge and Kegan Paul, 1971.

37. Apple D. How Laymen Define Illness. Journal of Health and Human Behaviour 1960. 1: 219-225.

38. Stoeckle J., Zola I. and Davidson G. On Going to see the Doctor: The Contribution of the Patient to the Decision to seek Medical Aid: A Selective Review. Journal of Chronic Diseases 1963; 16: 975-989.

39. Zola IK. Pathways to the Doctor: From Person to Patient. Social Science and Medicine 1972; 7: 677-689.

40. Mead M. Culture Health and Disease London: Tavistock, 1966.

41. Saunders L. Culture Differences and Medical Care New York: Russell Sage Foundation, 1954.

42. Zola IK. Culture and Symptoms: An Analysis of Patients Presenting Complaints. American Sociological Review 1960; 31: 613-630.

43. Hollingshead AB. and Redlich FC. Social Class and Mental Illness: A Community Study New York: Wiley, 1953.

44. Salloway JC. and Dillon PB. A Comparison of Family Relatives and Friends Networks in Health Care Utilization. Journal of Comparative Family Studies 1973; 4: 131-142.

45. Rosenstock TM. Why People use Health Services. Millbank Memorial Fund, Quarterly, 1966; 44: Part 2.

46. Zborowski M. Cultural Components in Responses to Pain. Journal of Social Issues 1952; 8: 16-30.

47. Shorter Oxford English Dictionary.

48. World Health Organization. Definition of Health from Preamble to the Constitution of the W.H.O. Basic Documents, 28th edition, Geneva: W.H.O., 1978, p.1.

49. Parsons T. Definitions of Health and Illness in Light of American Values and Social Structure on Patients, Physicians and Illness Ed. Jaco EG. (2nd edition.) New York: Free Press, 1972, 107-127.

50. Rossdale M. Health in a Sick Society. New Left Review 1965; 31: 82-90.

51. Dubos R. Man, Medicine and Environment

Harmondsworth: Penguin, 1970.

52. Wilson M. Health is for People London: Darton Longman and Todd Ltd., 1975.

53. Herzlich C. Opus Cit. p.19.

54. Dreitzel HP. (Ed.) The Social Organisation of Health Recent Sociology No. 3. New York: The Macmillan Co., 1971.

55. Brown GW. Social Causes of Disease. In Tuckett C. (Ed.) An Introduction to Medical Sociology London: Tavistock, 1976.

56. Kasl S. and Cobb S. Health Behaviour, Illness Behaviour and Sick-role Behaviour. Archives of Environmental Health 1966; 12: 246-266 and 531-541.

57. Koss E. The Health of Regionsville: What the People felt and did about it New York: Columbia Universities Press, 1954.

58. Foucault M. The Birth of the Clinic. An Archeology of Medical Perception London: Tavistock, 1973.

59. Rosenstock IM. The Health Belief Model and Preventive Health Behaviour. Health Education Monograph 1972; 2: 354-386.

60. Szasz TS. The Myth of Mental Illness London: Secker & Warburg, 1962.

61. Scheff TJ. Being Mentally Ill: A Sociological Theory Chicago: Aldine, 1966.

62. Shaw GB. The Doctor's Dilemma including Preface on Doctors Harmondsworth: Penguin, 1946. First produced as a play 1906.

63. Jeffreys M. Sociology and Medicine. Separation or Symbiosis. Lancet 1969; 1: 1111-1116.

64. Pflanz M. Sociology in Community Medicine. In Acheson RM. and Aird L. (Eds.) Seminars in Community Medicine Vol 1 Sociology London: Oxford University Press, 1976.

65. World Health Organisation. The Social Sciences in Medical Education. Report of a Seminar. Hanover 1969. Euro 0348, Copenhagen: W.H.O., 1970.

66. World Health Organisation. Report of the Working Group on the Social and Behavioural Sciences in Health Services and Manpower Development W.H.O., EMRO, 1977.

67. Susser MW. and Watson N. Sociology in Medicine London: Oxford University Press, 1971.

68. Balint M. The Doctor, His Patient and the Illness London: Tavistock Publication, 1964.

69. The Royal College of General Practitioners. The Future General Practitioners Learning and Teaching. British Medical Journal 1972.

70. Department of the Environment. Policy for

Inner Cities London: H.M.S.O., 1977. Cmnd 6845.

71. Donaldson RJ. Urban and Suburban Differentials. In Carter CO. and Peel J. (Eds.) Equalities and Inequalities in Health London: Academic Press, 1976.

72. Primary Health Care Study Group. Primary Health Care in Inner London A Report of a Study Group. London Health Planning Consortium, 1981.

73. Tuckett D. Work, Life-changes and Life Styles. In Tuckett D. (Ed.) An Introduction to Medical Sociology London: Tavistock, 1976, Chapter 4.

74. Rahe RH., Meyer M., Smith M. Kjaer G. and Holmes TH. Social Stress and Illness Onset. Journal of Psychosomatic Research 1964; 8: 35-44.

75. Taylor Lord and Chave S. Mental Health and Environment London: Longman, 1964.

76. Dohrenwend DS. and Dohrenwend BP. Social Status and Psychological Disasters. A Causal Inquiry New York: Wiley, 1979.

77. Holmes TH. and Rahe RH. The Social Readjustment Rating Scale. Journal of Psychosomatic Research 1967; 11: 213-218.

78. McEwen J. Health and Work. In Sutherland I. (Ed.) Health Education, Perspectives and Changes London: Allen & Unwin, 1979.

79. Parsons T. The Social System New York: The Free Press, 1951, Chapter 10.

80. Twaddle AG. Health Decisions and Sick Role Variations: An Explanation. Journal of Health and Social Behaviour 1969; 10: 105-115.

81. Gordon G. Role Theory and Illness; A Sociological Perspective New Haven: College and Unversity Press, 1966.

82. Lemert EM. Human Deviance , Social Problems and Social Control Englewood Cliffs, New Jersey: Prentice Hall, 1967.

83. Haber LD. and Smith RI. Disability as Deviance: Normative Adaptions of Role Behaviour. American Sociological Review 1971; 36: 87-97.

84. Illich I. Medical Nemesis. The Expropriation of Health London: Calder and Boyars, 1975. p.58-59.

85. Kosa J. and Zola IK. (Eds.) Poverty and Health: A Sociological Analysis Harvard: Harvard University Press, 1975.

86. Illich I. Opus Cit. p.167

87. Goffman E. Asylums Harmondsworth: Penguin, 1968.

88. Roth JA. Timetables Indianapolis: Bobbs-Merrill, 1963.

89. Davis F. <u>Passage Through Crisis</u> Indianapolis: Bobbs-Merrill, 1963.

90. Lemert EM. Opus Cit. p.50.

91. Szasz T. and Hollander MH. A Contribution to the Philosophy of Medicine. The Basic Models of Doctor-Patient Relationship. A.M.A. <u>Archives of Internal Medicine</u> 1956; 97: 585-592.

92. Howe G. Melvyn. Mortality from Selected Malignant Neoplasms in the British Isles: The Spatial Perspective. <u>Social Science & Medicine</u> 1981; 15D; No 1: 199-211.

93. Minter RE. Life Events and Illness Onset: A Review. <u>Psychosomatics</u> 1978; 19(6): 334-339.

94. Totman R. <u>Social Causes of Illness</u> London: Souvenier Press, 1979.

95. <u>Royal Commission on the National Health Service</u> Report (Merrison). London: H.M.S.O., 1979.

96. Department of Health and Social Security. <u>Priorities in the Health and Social Services. The Way Forward</u> London: H.M.S.O., 1977.

97. Department of Health and Social Security. <u>Care in Action. A Handbook of Policies and Priorities for the Health and Personal Social Services in England</u> London: H.M.S.O., 1981.

98. Navarro V. <u>Medicine Under Capitalism</u> London: Croom Helm, 1976. p.207-208.

99. Illich I. Opus Cit. p.168.

100. Navarro V. Opus Cit. p.93.

101. Mahler H. Health - A Demystification of Medical Technology. <u>Lancet</u> 1975; 2: 829-833.

102. Pill R. and Stott NCH. Concepts of Illness Causation and Responsibility: Some Preliminary Data from a Sample of Working Class Mothers. <u>Social Science and Medicine</u> 1982; 16: 43-52.

Chapter Five

PRIMARY CARE BEGINS AT HOME

> Fully 80% of illness is functional and can be
> effectively treated by any talented healer who
> displays warmth, interest and compassion
> regardless of whether he has finished grammar
> school. Another 10% of illness is wholly
> incurable. This leaves only 10% in which
> scientific medicine - at considerable cost - has
> any value at all. (1)

While many argue about the figures in the above
quotation, most people would agree that a
considerable proportion of illness is self-limiting
and that the main concern is to provide symptomatic
relief and simple general care. Equally in the much
smaller category - that of incurable illness, again,
the main concern is to provide symptomatic relief,
supportive care and attention. For both these
categories the majority of this treatment and care is
required in the home or the community setting.
Accordingly it is reasonable to consider the
contribution that the individual, family and
community make to health care. Self-medication is
probably one of the most important aspects of self-
care, as well as being one of the easiest to examine.
It exemplifies the relationship between self-care
and use of health services and illustrates the
importance of decision making by the patient and
family members.

Self medication has three main divisons: (i)
health promotion or health maintenance; (ii) treatment of trivial, self-limiting conditions or early
stages of more serious illness, and (iii) additional
care to that provided by health services in more
serious illness and in chronic conditions.

Generally, the first two occur with no reference
to the doctor or other health personnel. The largest

category is the second and this is related to the
widespread and frequent occurrence of symptoms.

THE CRAVING FOR MEDICATION

Sir William Osler, the great Canadian physician,
wrote at the end of the last century: "Man has an
inborn craving for medicine ... it is really one of
the most serious difficulties with which we have to
contend." (2)
    At about the same time, in England, Beatrice and
Sidney Webb (3) despite their concern and enthusiasm
for reform, opposed Lloyd George's 1911 National
Health Insurance Act, partly because of their fear
about the misuse of medication.

> Any such system (i.e. publicly subsidized
> systems with free choice of doctor) would lead,
> not only to a most serious increase upon the
> work and emoluments of the private practit-
> ioner, but also to an extravagant expenditure of
> public funds on popular remedies and 'medical
> extras', without obtaining in return for this
> enlarged medical relief, greater regularity of
> life or more hygienic habits in the patient.

    More recently, arguments have raged over the
question of prescription charges for prescribed
medicines in the National Health Service. To some, it
is a deterrent which discourages the unnecessary use
of prescribed medicine or indeed unnecessary visits
to general practitioners. It may also encourage
patients with minor, self-limiting conditions to
purchase their own over-the-counter products, rather
than seek a consultation and a prescription for the
same symptomatic remedy.
    However, various authors (4,5,6) reviewing the
subject of interaction between patient and doctor,
point to the complexity of patient and doctor
expectations of treatment. Although many patients
expect a prescription, there was little evidence to
support the often repeated professional comments
'that all the patient wants is a prescription'.
Frequently patient discontent is expressed when all
he or she gets from a consultation is a hurriedly
written prescription. Where therefore, does the
responsibility lie for the current enormous use -some
would say misuse - of both prescribed and over-the-
counter medicines - from the demands of the public -
or from the practitioners who too readily prescribe?

ROLE OF THE FAMILY

There has been a tendency in sociological literature
to debate whether or not traditional family functions
are being taken over increasingly by formal organizations with an emphasis on specialised skills. (7)
Adams (8) contends that "The medical function has
been transferred to the doctors' office and hospital"
and that "the home remedy, once the key element in
medical treatment, has become nothing more than the
butt of jokes."

Pratt (9) in a review which emphasized the
significance of the family in medication, considers
that the evidence does not support this with regard
to certain aspects of health care - particularly
self-medication. She believes that:

> the family's continued involvement in a
> specialised activity such as medication
> illustrates that the relationship between the
> family and specialised social systems is not
> adequately described by the concept of
> functional interdependence. The family and the
> health care system have their own distinctive
> interests and goals, which cause their
> relationships to include an element of power
> assertion and conflict. The family could not,
> therefore, safely delegate full responsibility
> for a critical task area such as medication to a
> specialised agency.

Pratt has shown the importance of health as
viewed by the family members.

> As an indication that families feel responsible
> for each others health, it was found in a sample
> of United States families that over half the
> wives and about four in ten husbands had worried
> about the health of other family members during
> the past week. More women listed family members'
> health as a source of worry than listed any of
> the other eight topics except bringing up
> children. When asked what they worried about
> most, 23% of the wives and 16% of the husbands
> listed health of family members.

Pratt concludes:

> Families distinctive interests, on the other
> hand, require that they assert a degree of
> control over medication that permits them to

53

assume full and timely servicing of members' health needs with minimum cost and bother, and protection of members from inappropriate and dangerous treatment by professionals. Insofar as families find that the restrictions on medication facilitate, or at least do not impede achievement of their own goals, the relationship between the family and the control agencies can be co-operative. However, it is not likely that restrictions designed to fulfil the objectives of professional groups and government agencies would conform in all respects to the needs of families, with their distinctive goals and responsibilities. And it may become even less likely because the family must assume greater responsibility, rather than less, to discriminatingly select, co-ordinate and evaluate, and manage the complex variety of medications and other therapies required by family members. The tendency of the medical care system to become increasingly technical, internally specialised and bureaucratized has rendered it less capable of providing overall co-ordination and management of medication for individuals and families. Thus, the relationship between the health care system and the family include an essential element of manipulation, power assertion, and conflict, as well as functional reciprocity.

Indeed, there is evidence of the increasing role of the family in self-care despite some of the influences to the contrary. An holistic (10) approach encourages an individual and a family role in health; the reduction of hospitalisation, the provision of facilities for parents to be in hospital with their children; pressure by families to be involved in mental health; the possibility of intermittent hospital and home care; and wider provision of day-care facilities. All this tends to increase links between professionals and families and requires to be based on co-operation and understanding of roles and needs, the differing contributions and the limitations of both.

SYMPTOMS AND ILLNESS IN THE COMMUNITY

As indicated in a previous chapter, feeling unwell is a common experience. Many different community studies in a wide range of countries have shown the

54

extent of symptoms and illness. These have often been
expressed in different ways.

At first sight, it would appear that there is a
contradiction between people's estimate of their
state of health and the presence of health
complaints. Wadsworth and his colleagues, (11) when
they asked their study-population, the question,
"Would you say that your state of health during the
last fourteen days was perfect, good, fair or poor?",
found that 35% of respondents assessed their state of
health as 'perfect', 34% felt that they were in
'good' health, 21% said their health was 'fair', and
10% felt in 'poor' health. However, in only 4.9% were
no health complaints reported. Therefore, the fact
that an individual has experienced some symptom or
complaint did not mean that this was not compatible
with 'good' or even a 'perfect' state of health. This
clearly indicates that acute, and self-limiting
conditions are regarded as normal.

Other community studies have shown similar
results. Logan and Brooke (12) in an earlier study
found slightly lower figures - 76% of women and 67%
of men reported some illness during the month prior
to interview. Bell and her colleagues (13,14) in a
new town in Scotland, reported that over a three week
period 94% of the study population of women
experienced some illness symptoms.

15% reported 1 symptom
59% reported between 2 and 5 symptoms
20% reported 5 or more symptoms
The mean was 3.06 per woman.

Dunnell and Cartwright (15) sum up the situation
by stating that the majority of a population report
at least one symptom during a two week period (5% of
adults are symptom free - the average reported number
of symptoms are 3.9, but it was 6.2 among those who
said that their health was poor and in contrast it
was 2.5 for those reporting excellent health. More
children - 37% were symptom free.)

An alternative way to examine this is to
consider the cumulative experience of an individual.
An American study (16) has shown that acute illnesses
requiring reduced activity or medical attention are
experienced at the rate of 2 per person per year.
During a twenty year period the average lower middle
class man between 20 and 45 years experiences
approximately 1 life endangering illness, 20
disabling experiences, 200 non-disabling illnesses
and 1,000 symptomatic episodes. (17) That is, a total

of 1,221 episodes or one new episode every six days.

In a detailed study using health diaries Morrell and Wale (18) found that women in the age group 20-44 years recorded a symptom of illness on 1 day in 3. It is likely that the use of health diaries will result in more accurate recording of symptoms. Records as used in most studies may underestimate symptoms. By taking account of the family or household the frequency of illness and symptoms becomes even more apparent. In a study of 273 households over a 30 week period, (19) there was an average of 12.4 acute illnesses or injuries per family averaging 57.4 total illness days per household. An average family experiences and copes with illness on 1 day in 4.

Although much of this is related to acute and self-limiting conditions some of these symptoms result from chronic conditions, and an American Government Survey (20) has reported that half of the civilian population of the United States have one or more chronic conditions.

From these studies it appears that most families deal almost continually with symptoms and illness. Most of their symptoms are rather vague and general. Bell and her colleagues (13,14) reported the following breakdown of complaints:

Tiredness, feeling run down	60%
Headache	49%
Backache	29%
Colds	27%
Coughs	24%
Skin Trouble	20%

Relating complaints to disease classification, Wadsworth and his colleagues (11) found that the commonest system affected was the respiratory system followed by mental and psycho-neurotic disorder and the bones and organs of movement (see Table 5.1).

ACTION TAKEN

Self-care is the true first level of health care and comprises numerically the major portion of the system. There are more people caring for their own complaints than there are attending health professionals. Self-care taking place within the family context dictates to a degree the whole pattern of health care. The better and more effective that self-care becomes the less, in theory, will be the need to utilize medical resources. (21)

The overall relationship between self-care, primary care as provided by the general practitioners or other first-line health professionals and specialist or hospital care is shown in Figure 5.1. Figure 5.2 summarises the action that is taken by patients when they experience symptoms. As far as a general practice population is concerned, in a typical practice of 2,500 in a given year, about 70% of the patients will visit their general practitioner at least once. About 17% of these will be referred to outpatients and about 10% will be admitted to hospital. (22) Table 5.2, taken from Wadsworth's study (11) shows the relative significance of the patient and doctor in diagnosing different conditions. This close relationship is also apparent when the conditions presenting to general practitioners and the symptoms which are self treated are examined. (Tables 5.3 and 5.4). It is interesting to note that an analysis of conditions presented to occupational health services (23) shows a very similar pattern. (Table 5.5).

Morrell and Wale (18) compared the symptoms recorded in the health diary and those presented to the doctor, and although the broad categories are similar, they concluded that the patients were very discriminating in deciding what to present to the doctor. They suggest that as few as 1 in 37 symptoms may be referred to the general practitioners when full details of symptom experience, as recorded in health diaries are examined.

Overall, 18% of symptoms led to a restriction of activities and 57% to medication - usually non-prescribed.

Medication

Most studies have examined the entire subject of medication and have compared and contrasted the prescribed and the non-prescribed components. These studies have generally shown a greater proportion of non-prescribed medicines, both kept in the house and used by individuals. Variations in use are found in different countries, socially and culturally distinct communities and age groups.

Medicines in the House

The stocks of medicines held in a home, and the purchasing of medicines provides a useful indicator of families' preparedness for coping with illness as well as showing their previous experience with medication. Dunnell and Cartwright (15) found an average of 7.3 non-prescription and 3.0 prescription medicines in a household. Knapp and Knapp (24) in the United States found higher figures of 17.2 non-prescription and 5.3 prescription medicines per household.

They noted that during a 30 week study period the mean number of drugs procured was 13.7 and that 95% of the households procured at least one drug. Roney and Nall (25) in the United States reported similarly high figures and in a two week study period found that 86 families purchased 154 medications of which 94 were over-the-counter preparations selected by the families themselves.

In Britain, most households have immediate access to some home medication - 91% having one or more medicines in the household. (15) Nearly all had analgesics and skin cream, 1/5th had sedatives, tranquillisers or sleeping pills and 2/5ths had one or more items that the informant could not identify. (This last piece of information indicates a potentially hazardous situation which will be discussed later).

Self-care for minor injury is another important aspect and a survey in the United States (26) found that 90% of houses kept the basic elements for treating minor injury - bandages, adhesive plasters, gauze and cotton wool.

Another indication of the amount of medicine available in homes has resulted from campaigns, usually carried out by health education authorities to collect 'surplus' or 'unused' medicines. These medicines are primarily prescribed - up to 90%. This may indicate that non-prescribed medicines are retained and not disposed of. Frequently prescribed medicines, long out of date, no longer available or deteriorated through age or poor storage, are collected. 44% of medicines were kept in the kitchen, 23% in the bathroom, 29% of self-prescribed had been in the house for one year or more and 1 in 5 had not been used in the past year. (15)

More recently in a survey of households in England and Wales (27) the average home was found to have 3.2 containers of prescribed medicine - 56% were in current use, 16% in occasional use, and 28% were never used. One fifth of all oral antibiotics found in the study were wasted. A rough estimate suggests that £23m. of prescription products (5.6% of the total) are wasted annually in England and Wales.

Prescribed and Non Prescribed

Most studies have reported approximately twice as much use of non-prescribed medicines as prescribed medicines and this seems to have remained fairly constant during the last twenty years.

Jeffreys and her colleagues (28) in a new housing area in 1960 reported during a one month study period that one quarter of their population had taken prescribed medicines, while two thirds had taken non-prescribed. Dunnell and Cartwright (15) reported during a two week period that 41% of adults had used prescribed and 67% non-prescribed drugs. Hannay (29) in a study in Glasgow found almost the same number of people on prescribed as taking unprescribed – approximately one third but in fact more prescribed medicines were being taken as there were individuals taking several prescribed medicines at one time. Bell and her colleagues (13,14) in a Scottish new town found 79% taking non-prescribed compared with 21% on medicines prescribed by the general practitioner.

In an extensive international study Kohn and White (30) found the highest rates of medication in the United States of America and Canada, where up to 75% of the populations studied were on medication – 40% being self-medication. The lowest rates were in Poland and Yugoslavia – 28% on medication – 10% being self-medication. There is considerable stability of patterns within countries. Use of medication tends to increase with age and be higher for females than males. In all study areas vitamins form a substantial percentage. In summary they conclude that in most study areas there is substantial self-medication and even use of medicines whose contributions to health seems doubtful. Overall use of medicines tends to be high, perhaps even disproportionate in relationship to levels of perceived morbidity and chronicity, and there is the suggestion that consumption of at least non-prescribed medicines may be directly related to economic descriptors of relative financial affluence.

The Nature of the Medication

As already indicated by Hannay's study (29) many people were on more than one medication and sometimes there is a combination of prescribed and non-prescribed drugs. In over 68% of episodes only non-prescribed are used. (24) In Bell's Scottish study (13,14) it was found that 40% had taken one medication, 39% between two and five, and 1% more than five types of medication.

Although there have been some variations in definitions in the studies, particularly regarding analgesics and antipyretics which form the major category of self-medication (up to 50%), the following tables from Dunnell and Cartwright (15) and Wadsworth and his colleagues (11) illustrate the overall picture (Tables 5.6 and 5.7). Crooks and Christopher (31) in a study of those purchasing medicines in a chemist shop, found that analgesics headed the list with 27%, antacids 12%, laxatives 9%, antitussives 8% and expectorants 7%. Benylin was the single most popular at 4.4%. There were eight analgesics among the top twelve preparations of which four contained multiple ingredients. Paracetemol was the commonest active ingredient. Approximately 12% of the items contained anti-histamines – cough medicines, nasal decongestants and travel sickness remedies. The reasons for choosing the particular medicines were – own assessment in 31%, advice from the chemist in 21%, and doctor's advice in 14%. There was little evidence of influence from the media – newspapers 2%, T.V. 2%. One purchaser was found to be taking four types of analgesic tablet, three of which contained paracetemol and was taking a total of seventeen tablets per day. The symptoms most likely to lead to self-medication are temperature 94%, headache 83%, indigestion 81%, sore throat 78%. (15) In the Glasgow study (29) 79% of analgesics and antipyretics were not prescribed.

Although aspirin and pain killers were the commonest medication in adults, in children skin ointments and antiseptics were the commonest self-treatments (or more correctly parent treatments). (15)

In a study of a small self-contained community, Jones (32) was able to gain additional information on self-medication by simultaneous recording of doctor-patient contacts and chemist sales. This showed as most other studies have, that twice as many people went to the chemist to buy their own medicine as consulted the doctor, but that there were variations with the different symptom complexes examined. People were more content to treat their own symptoms of coughs, colds and indigestion, than they were to treat diarrhoea and sickness, and apparently claimed more success. The number of people asking the chemist's advice before purchase was much higher than reported in other studies and may reflect the high esteem which the chemist had in that particular community.

The possible scope of self-medication is seen by the number of preparations which are available. Martindales' Extra Pharmacopoeia (33) lists over 1,400 preparations of which 8% contain multiple ingredients.

Few studies have described the contribution of traditional or home remedies. Eliott-Binns (34) found that home remedies (those which traditionally came from the kitchen, household or garden) accounted for 15% of all advice given by the lay system. Female relatives advised them more frequently than male relatives, while the widowed and separated used them more often than the married. They were recommended progressively more frequently by the older age groups except that teenagers advised them more often than expected. The acceptance rate for home remedies was less than for medicines. Bell and her colleagues (13,14) found little use of traditional medicine, but this may have been related to the special social characteristics and the lack of social networks in a new town.

Self-medication may be a form of care on its own, it may be a prelude to contact with the general practitioner, or it may co-exist. International studies have indicated that approximately half of the patients attending for primary care by doctors had previously self-medicated. That this applies to the earlier stages of more serious conditions is indicated by the fact that approximately 40% of patients attending an out-patient clinic had tried treating themselves initially. Danaher and her colleagues (35,36) in a London study suggested that those who attended general practitioners for a particular symptom, tended to self-treat for an insufficient period of time before consultation compared with non-attenders with the same symptoms even though the severity of the symptom was similar. Overall, those who had taken self-prescribed medicines for symptoms were less likely to consult a doctor. Figures for co-existing treatment of prescribed and non-prescribed range from 10-30%.

Many medicines are taken over a long period of time. Crooks and Christopher (31) in their study of those purchasing over-the-counter medicines in a pharmacy found that 21% had been taking it for six months or more, and that long continued use was common in the elderly - 57% in those 65 years or over, compared with 29% in the whole group. Clearly there is a greater possibility of habitual use and this was related to antacids, analgesics and laxatives.

One factor which emerges repeatedly from studies is that women dose themselves more than men. (37) We can only speculate about the reasons for this. (15) Perhaps it is to do with the feeling that women can less easily take to their beds than men and so are more anxious to ward off illness. Perhaps it is because women do more shopping and so over-the-counter drugs are more easily available. Perhaps women actually do suffer more from ailments amenable to self-medication or make greater use of social networks, which give more advice on diverse approaches to treatment, encouraging self-care.

Those Who Did Nothing

It is perhaps interesting to comment briefly on this group. Wadsworth and his colleagues (11) reported that no action had been taken by 18.8% of respondents with health problems. While some of this may be accounted for by acute, very short lived conditions, Bell (13,14) in her study found that for certain more chronic conditions, action might also not be taken. 50% of those who felt run down and 81% of those with backache did nothing. While it is only possible to speculate as to the reason, it may be that these conditions are accepted 'as part of life'. As Festinger (38) has pointed out, when people believe that they cannot change a situation they often come to believe that it is satisfactory, because it is only in this way that they can get rid of the sense of worry and unease arising from the wish to change something which they think is unchangeable.

NORMAL USE

In a fascinating paper, Blum (39) has drawn attention to "Normal Drug Use". As he pointed out, while concern is frequently expressed over the 'abuse' of psychoactive drugs, little is known of the normal or non-abusive use of such substances. Different countries, cultures and religions have views on the use of varying substances to modify behaviour, feeling or function. Legal restrictions in some countries prevent the purchase of alcohol below a certain age, in some countries it is banned altogether: other countries permit alcohol use, but prohibit the use of cannabis. Table 5.8 summarises one part of Blum's findings.

The study has also examined the pattern of drug usage, the relationship between different categories of drugs, and related those to social and personal factors.

One finding was that persons with greater drug experience had more experience of medical care, believed in the efficacy of medication and gave drugs to others as well as self-medicating to a greater extent.

HEALTH PROMOTING APPROACHES

Studies in the United States and Britain (28,40,41,42) have indicated that there is considerable interest in health promoting activities - although much of this could not be described as self-medication, it is generally believed that 'good' nutrition is most important and that a major reason for ill health is poor, improper or inadequate nutrition. For both adults and children, vitamins form an important aspect of this health promoting activity. During the 1970's the interest in healthy eating developed greatly. This occured in two main directions. Firstly, an interest in health foods, a move away from modern packaged convenience foods to older, simpler and often cheaper substitutes. Sometimes this is associated with a particular organization or philosophy, while sometimes it is related to other attempts to improve the quality of life or escape from conventional society. Secondly, at a medical or scientific level, there has been discussion of the merits and risks of certain foods or patterns of eating. Frequently the evidence has been limited or conflicting - cholesterol, polyunsaturated fats and fibre. As there is the possibility of developing a national nutritional policy and as there are implications for health education, it is important to try and disentangle the evidence from the various commercial interests. (43)

TAKING PRESCRIBED MEDICINES

Not only do patients decide when to seek professional advice, but also in association with the advice of family, friends and colleagues, they make decisions about taking the treatment that has been prescribed. This may range from not completing the prescribed course, through altering the dosage, or the directions, to keeping some of the prescribed medicines for future use, giving it to someone else, or seeking to continue treatment by means of repeat prescriptions, either with or without direct consultation with the doctor. Alteration of dosage, or cessation of treatment before the prescribed course is completed is usually labelled by doctors as non-compliance, (44) but it may indicate purposeful cessation because of side effects (perhaps not adequately explained at the time the treatment was prescribed at consultation), or improvement of the conditions (the necessity for completing a course of antibiotics even if the patient feels better, is not always explained fully or understood).

Any comprehensive examination of compliance mentions terms such as attitudes, information, education, communication, relationships and management. And the problem is related to the type of medication or the social and cultural environment. The title of a recent review "Patient Compliance: A Multifaceted Problem With No Easy Solution" (45) seems to summarise current knowledge.

Dunnell and Cartwright (15) summarised the position: 2.5% of prescriptions are not filled at all; 16% are thrown away before being used up and 20% are not taken as directed.

A review of 68 studies of patients' compliance with advice showed that on average 44% of patients did not follow the advice given to them. (46) Some studies (47,48) in specialised problems have indicated considerable under-use of prescribed medicine. Even in hospital where nurses handed out the tablets, there was substantial rejection by schizophrenic patients. In an ante-natal clinic it was reported that 32% had stopped taking iron. Linnett (49) has postulated that there is only a 50% chance of the drugs prescribed in general practice being taken but this is higher than suggested by other studies.

A slighty different aspect of medication that is primarily under the control of the patients is the 'repeat prescription'. This represents a sizeable aspect of patient requests for care in general practice. Manasse (50) found that the number of prescriptions requested (during a one month study period) was 37 per 1,000, this representing 50 items per 1,000 patients. The majority of these represented routine requests (81.9%) followed by sporadic treatment (10.4%) such as seasonal antihistamines and topical steroids. About 30% of all requests were for psychiatric drugs. An interesting aspect of 'repeat prescribing' is the apparent increase in the number of those prescriptions that are obtained via the receptionist and do not involve direct contact with the general practitioner. (51) Madeley (52) found that 52% of all prescriptions in the study practice in London were repeats - 38% arising in consultations with the doctor and 22% through the receptionist. This overall figure of repeat prescriptions is higher than that recorded by Dunnell and Cartwright (15) in 1972 - 25% and Balint et al in 1970, 41%.

There is obviously a very large variation between different practices and although the attitude of the general practitioners is a most important factor, the attitudes and actions of patients is also likely to make a significant contribution. Balint and his colleagues (53) examined the characteristics of the 'Repeat-prescription patients':

The chief characteristics were: the long-repeat patients tend to marry earlier than the rest of the population but they also have a much greater tendency to become secondarily single (widowed, separated, or divorced) earlier; they make contact with their doctor more frequently than the others, but see to it that this contact is, on the whole, not too intimate. Thus they ask for a home visit only slightly more frequently than the rest, but use 'indirect contacts' more than twice as often (by 'indirect contact' we mean letters, telephone calls, or sending a messenger such as a spouse, child, parent, or other relative, friend or neighbour for the prescription). To explain these ambivalent attitudes, we formed the hypothesis that the balance between gratifications and frustrations in the life of long-repeat patients is unfavourable, creating tensions and strains in them which they experience as unpleasant bodily sensations; they feel that they need 'something' and go to their doctors to 'complain'. As a rule, no physical or chemical examination - however subtle and sensitive - can find any localizable illness in them. In consequence, the doctor, trained in illness-centred medicine, cannot achieve much with his professional knowledge and skill. Nevertheless, he goes on trying, as is shown by the much higher incidence of multiple diagnoses in the long-repeat group.
In spite of all this effort, no satisfactory diagnosis can be established and, in consequence, no rational therapy devised.

The patient continues to come and to complain in search of the 'something' that he feels he needs, but remains unsatisfied - the doctor tries hard but cannot achieve reliable and durable results; in this way a strained relationship develops between the two. Then the repeat prescription is introduced and the situation changes for the better: a good deal of strain in their relationship disappears; its place is taken by insincere mutual appreciation based not on reality but on overvaluation. The patient accepts the drug as the symbol of his 'something' and demands, as a rule, that his drug should remain for ever 'good, reliable, unchanging and always available'. The doctor feels uneasy - he knows that he does not deserve the praise and appreciation but accepts them because they help to preserve the peace. Some doctors are even proud of their ability to help patients in this way; the majority, however, are embarrassed, try to excuse themselves, to minimise the number of repeat prescriptions in their practice, to put the blame for initiating them on everybody but themselves.

Recently, Mapes (54) in his study of patient prescribing has drawn attention to the apparent increase in the number of repeat prescriptions obtained through the receptionist (or practice staff other than the general practitioner). The term 'apparent' is used because this is indicated by the different 'hands' on the prescription. It would seem that this aspect of continued medication which is primarily being initiated by the patient is an area that would repay study, to examine the knowledge, attitudes, satisfaction and dissatisfaction of both patients and doctors.

SAFETY AND RISKS

In any medication there are a number of possible risks. With prescribed drugs, an error may be made by the prescribing doctor or pharmacist - the wrong drug may be issued or the directions may be inappropriate - this is rare. (55) The patient may take the wrong medicine especially if there are a large number of old, similar looking medicines in the household or may take it in a dangerous and ineffective manner. This may be the result of accident, personal confusion or purposeful intent. Inappropriate dosage is a greater risk with children. There may be interaction between drugs prescribed and unprescribed and food or alcohol. Drugs may have deteriorated through age and/or incorrect storage.

A study described in a letter to the Lancet revealed widespread ignorance and confusion about the purposes and dangers of antibiotics among patients and some nurses. (56) Another study showed that only 50% of people read the labels on drugs. (57) The interaction of drugs is an extremely complicated field. Interaction can reduce or enhance the effect of the drug or even be dangerous to the patient. (58) A further cause for anxiety about self-medication was thrown up in a survey of self-medication in a small community; namely, that it could conceal symptoms of a serious illness. (32) There seems to be quite a high level of awareness by the public of possible side effects - this is particularly so in pregnancy where the disasterous effects of thalidomide are still well remembered and there is general caution about medicines during pregnancy. The possible ill effects of artificial sweeteners and the widely publicised brain damage attributed to vaccination are recent reminders.

Although at present most attention is linked to the side effects of prescribed drugs, it is useful to remember that some of the over-the-counter preparations can also have undesirable and sometimes serious ill effects. Pink disease, (59,60) erythroedema or acrodynia, as it was called, is an interesting example of a condition quite common in the 1930's but now extinct. It was the result of chronic mercurial poisoning from teething powders which were freely available in chemists and grocery shops throughout the country. Currently, the possible serious side effects of certain remedies used by some immigrant communities in Britain have been highlighted. (61) One of them, bal-jivan chamcho, bears a striking similarity to the mercurial teething powders, but the metal involved is usually lead and originates from the spoon containing the child's medicine. Remedies used by Hakims and other practitioners of the Unani and Areyuvidic systems of medicine frequently contain metallic substances, modern drugs and herbal remedies. The risks of lead containing surma (62), used as a cosmetic, and treatment for certain eye conditions have been noted in children.

Two important recent reminders of possible serious side effects of over-the-counter preparations are kidney damage from the analgesic, phenacetin, and the problem of subacute myeloptic neuropathy, resulting from clioquinol (enterovioform). The large number of substances - prescribed drugs, laxatives, oral contraceptives, industrial solvents, herbs and contaminated cereals which may cause liver damage illustrate the complexity and with a time lag in some cases to produce the ill-effects, it may be very difficult to trace what caused the problem. (63)

There is relatively little definitive information about side effects from non-prescribed drugs. Crooks and Christopher (31) found that 6.6% of those purchasing over-the-counter preparations (including first-time users) had experienced a side effect to that particular product (or similar medicant) and overall 7.3% know of side effects.

So, on the grounds of safety, should self-medication be discouraged? The answer seems to be, on balance, 'no'.

Firstly, the worries about drug complexities can be alleviated to some extent by the operation of stringent controls over powerful drugs being sold over the counter and by detailed instructions, but who makes decisions as to which drugs to sell? Pharmaceutical companies have a serious responsibility for the safety of their products. (64) One commentator suggests that Oxytetracycline (an antibiotic) should be sold, with full instructions, over the counter. (65) Would this lead to unnecessary or even harmful use? In many countries of the world, antibiotics, steroids and many other powerful drugs are easily available. By limiting powerful drugs to prescriptions, the patient is unfortunately not protected from their abuse. It was found in the United States of America that 95% of doctors would issue prescriptions for coughs and colds - (although most British doctors believe coughs and colds are suitable for self-medication) - of which 60% would be antibiotics. (66) This pointer to antibiotic-happy doctors is reinforced in a guide to medicines for lay people, by Parish (67) who says that the risks:

> ... apply to both prescription and over-the-counter drug preparations. The intervention of a doctor may not necessarily offer protection for the consumer. It is a sad fact that a high proportion of adverse drug effects caused by prescription drugs could have been predicted and prevented by prescribing doctors. These dangers are increased because poor communication between doctor, pharmacist and patient

often leaves the consumer in almost total ignorance of the benefits and risks of any drug preparation he takes.

Which seems to bring us back to the point mentioned previously, that perhaps the best way patients can be protected is for them to have the knowledge and to be able to partake in the decisions. A patient knowing he or she is allergic to penicillin, will be able to tell this to anyone providing treatment. If it is hidden away in the medical notes it might easily be missed.

These few examples appear to be the exception rather than the rule, and from the standpoint of assessment by doctors (36) of the effectiveness and safety of self-medication, there is general agreement that it is safe, appropriate and unlikely to lead to delay in presenting to doctors the more serious problems. This last concern is most frequently voiced. (68) The risk of interaction between self-medication, prescribed drugs and food or alcohol is a real but probably small problem. Williamson and Danaher (35) summarise professional attitudes to self-medication in Tables 5.9 and 5.10.

General practitioners asked to assess the self-treatment of a particular group, judged it to be partially or completely effective in 75% of cases and potentially harmful in only 5%. There is obviously room for continued improvement and review. The literature on self-medication indicates that there is a broad consensus that with this new recognition of the extent and worth of self-medication comes a responsibility for the professionals to share their knowledge and make the self-care informed and intelligent.

SUMMARY OF PRESENT POSITION

So self-medication is not a fringe activity, not a new idea. It is the normal 'common-sense' way of behaving when dealing with an illness. What is new is the revival of interest and the official recognition now being given to self-care and old fashioned remedies. Traditional medicines and alternative approaches to health maintenance and care are being accorded a new respectability by bodies such as the World Health Organization, and old remedies are being revived and evaluated. There is a new enthusiasm for herbal treatments, attributable perhaps to the interest in the natural environment and a creeping disillusionment with modern medicine. The Herbal Society receives increasing support in its search for new remedies, (69) and in its review of long established and popular treatments on health promoting substances.

But to turn from the global to the individual. Why do people self-medicate instead of going to the doctor? Perhaps in these days of free medical service the fact that the public still consumes twice as many over-the-counter, as prescribed, drugs, does require some explanation.

Why Do People Self-Medicate?

1. The illness is trivial. Although there is evidence from Dunnell and Cartwright (15) that 25% of all general practitioner consultations are unnecessary, it seems that in the majority of cases, people can distinguish between serious and trivial disease. For instance, 96% of women interviewed for a study, said they would go to the doctor for unusual bleeding or discharge whereas only 8% of people said they would go for dandruff. (70) 80% of those prescribing over-the-counter medicines thought the illness too trivial to matter to the general practitioner. Even though a perfect balance can never be achieved, not least because the professionals themselves are ambivalent, there is not a great deal of controversy in the majority of conditions between public and professional. One faction deplores self-care on the grounds that any slight symptom may herald a serious complaint. The other encourages it on the grounds that people should not bother the doctor with every minor complaint. (65)

2. Wasting the doctor's time. Not only is the patient's perception of the disease relevant but also the doctor's - real or imagined. Even though a patient believes a disease might be serious, he or she is concerned that the doctor will see it as trivial and consider the patient to be wasting his or her time. (70)

3. Nothing can be done. This is applicable to both (supposedly) chronic - ("there's no cure for rheumatism so I'll just have to put up with it") -and fatal - ("this lump means cancer, so there's no point in going to the doctor") illnesses. The degree to which people are prepared to put up with complaints without seeking alleviation is illustrated in a study to investigate what people did about their skin diseases. It was found that only 27% of those with moderate or severe ezcema sought professional

help. (71)

4. <u>Fear of repercussions of diagnosis</u>. The mother at home may fear being told to go to bed, if there is no-one to care for the children, while the breadwinner fears being told to stay off work, which means for most families, a cut in their income by half. Because doctors feature prominently in our social definitions of sickness, patients may avoid the surgery since it is possible to ignore sickness and its implications only so long as it remains officialy undiagnosed.

5. <u>Poor experiences of doctors leading to lack of faith</u>. This is linked with non-compliance, in that both non-compliance and non-attendance can result from the undermining of confidence in the doctor caused by a real or apparent, lack of interest in the patient or the ailment. Doctors write out prescriptions before they have even heard the problem. Depressed patients who want only to talk are given pills they don't want. (66) Ryan describes examples from the Soviet Union where lack of faith, or alternative advice led to self-medication. (72)

6. <u>Inconvenience</u>. The Office of Health Economics ran a series of group discussions to determine attitudes to medication and found that people would go to the chemist rather than return to the doctor, for repeat medicines because: "Time is important to most people. The thought of a long spell in a crowded waiting room inhibits many people from making a visit to their doctor." (70) Similarly, the skin survey mentioned above found that although, in the case of eczema, self-medication was more expensive and less effective, its easy availablility outweighed these disadvantages. (71)

Self-medication, although it is an easily recognisable entity is not something separate from the wider field of self-care and its intimate relationship with other health related activities - must be recognised. In both self-treatment and in health prevention, people may indulge in other activities which are considered to help achieve the desired aim - alteration in diet, more or less exercise, taking a rest, having a holiday, reduction in work, warmth, fresh air, bread poultices and so on.

It must be remembered that alcohol and other substances may be used to achieve the same purposes - some aspects of the normal use of medicines may be very similar to the normal use of alcohol - the gin and tonic for relaxation after a hard day at the office, the nightcap to encourage sleep or the glass of tonic wine for the person feeling a 'little run down'.

Self-medication is a normal and appropriate part of the overall provision of health care. This is recognised by professionals who equally recognise that the general practitioner could not cope if self-care was to be abolished. New educational roles for professionals are suggested which in turn would involve change in curricula in professional education and training. New participation for patients is proposed which would result in an alteration in the traditional patient-professional relationship. There is a need to re-examine policy to see what resources are required to achieve their aims and to determine methods of evaluating any changes which are implemented.

FIGURE 5.1:   Extent of Self-Care

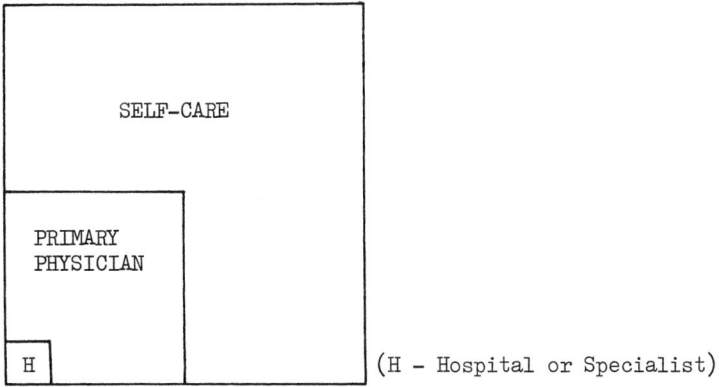

(From: Fry, 1978)

FIGURE 5.2:   Actions for Symptoms Information

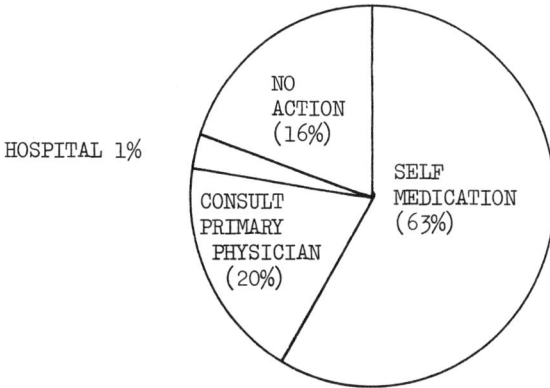

from Logan and Brooke, 1957; Jeffreys et al., 1960;
Wadsworth et al., 1971; Dunnell and Cartwright, 1982.

(From: Fry, 1978)

TABLE 5.1

All reported active complaints by ISC
(4-digit) classification in rank order

ISC classification	No.	%
Respiratory system	2,397	25.7
Mental, psychoneurotic, etc. disorders	1,968	21.1
Bones and organs of movement	1,433	15.4
Digestive system	1,012	10.9
Nervous system and sense organs	719	7.7
Skin and cellular tissue	502	5.4
Circulatory system	393	4.2
Accidents	316	3.4
Ill-defined conditions	212	2.3
Genito-urinary system	208	2.2
Congenital malformation	71	0.8
Infective and parasitic disease	60	0.6
Pregnancy and complications	13	0.1
Allergic, endocrine, metabolic and nutritional disease	10	0.1
Neoplastic disease	1	0.01
Total	9,315	100.0

From: Wadsworth, Butterfield and Blaney, 1971.

TABLE 5.2

Complaints according to who had
originally made the diagnosis

Rank Order	ISC Disease Category	Who Diagnosed Doctor	Who Diagnosed Respondent	Total (100%)
1	Respiratory system	37.0	63.0	2,397
2	Mental, psychoneurotic, etc.	19.6	80.4	1,968
3	Bones and organs of movement	39.2	60.8	1,433
4	Digestive sysem	22.7	77.3	1,012
5	Nervous system and sense organs	40.9	59.1	719
6	Skin and cellular tissue	27.3	72.7	502
7	Circulatory system	42.0	58.0	383
8	Accidents	22.0	78.0	316
9	Symptoms and senility NEC*	27.4	72.6	212
10	Genito-urinary system	23.6	76.4	208
11	Congenital malformation	85.9	14.1	71
12	Infective and parasitic disease	58.3	41.7	60
13	Pregnancy and complications	100.0	-	13
14	Allergic and endocrine disease	70.0	30.0	10
15	Neoplastic disease	100.0	-	1
	Total	32.0	68.0	9,315

*NEC means throughout 'not elsewhere classified'

(From: Wadsworth, Butterfield and Blaney)

TABLE 5.3

Percentages of groups of conditions
in primary care (from Fry, 1974)

Groups of Conditions	per cent
Common respiratory infections	25
Emotional, nervous or psychiatric disorders	15
Gastro-intestinal disorders	10
Skin disorders	10
Non-illness	10
Others	30

(From: Fry 1978)

TABLE 5.4

Percentages of common groups of symptoms
self-treated (from Dunnell and Cartwright, 1972)

Symptoms	per cent
Respiratory Coughs, colds, catarrh, flu, sore throats	25
Rheumatic Aches and pains in joints, backache, painful feet	20
Emotional and Nervous Anxiety, depression, tiredness, headaches	20
Gastro-intestinal Indigestion, bowel disturbances	10
Skin disorders Rashes	5
Others Accidents, cardio-vascular, gynaecological, eye problems, etc.	20

(From: Fry, 1978)

TABLE 5.5

The relationship of the diagnosis to the rate of return to work
and other disposals (%) following contact with Occupational Health Services

		Disposal (%)			
Diagnostic groupings	Return to work end of shift	Home	Not at work	Hosp /G.P.	Total no with diagnosis
Infectious diseases	96.3	0.3	2.4	0.3	295
Neoplasms	0.0	100.0	0.0	0.0	1
Allergic, endocrine, metabolic diseases	91.7	5.6	0.9	1.9	108
Diseases of blood and blood forming organs	100.0	0.0	0.0	0.0	1
Mental disorders	80.3	14.8	0.0	3.3	61
Diseases of the nervous system	85.9	13.1	0.0	0.0	99
Diseases of the eye	97.4	0.2	0.3	1.5	612
Diseases of the ear	97.4	0.6	0.9	0.3	340
Diseases of the circulatory system	72.7	19.0	0.8	5.8	121
Upper respiratory tract infections	95.1	3.8	0.3	0.0	1,660
Other respiratory diseases	84.4	9.9	2.8	2.1	141
Diseases of the mouth and teeth	93.3	3.1	0.5	1.5	195
Disorders of function of stomach	86.0	13.0	0.4	0.4	897
Other diseases of digestive system	93.5	6.5	0.0	0.0	31
Dysmenorrhoea	90.6	9.4	0.0	0.0	127
Diseases of urinary system	82.2	15.6	0.0	0.0	45
Diseases of genital system	63.2	36.8	0.0	0.0	19
Complications of pregnancy and puerperium	60.0	33.3	0.0	6.7	15
Rash and ill-defined skin conditions	96.1	3.4	0.0	0.0	204
Other diseases of skin	96.8	1.0	1.0	0.8	1,079
Pain in back	95.3	3.6	0.5	0.5	193
Pain in joint	95.9	2.0	0.1	1.0	98
Other pain	90.1	7.0	0.0	2.8	71
Other diseases of musculo-skeletal system	91.1	3.3	3.9	0.6	180
Congenital abnormalities	100.0	0.0	0.0	0.0	1
Headache	96.2	2.9	0.4	0.3	762
Other symptoms and ill-defined conditions	71.2	25.0	3.0	0.0	132
Personal problems	91.3	7.2	1.4	0.0	69
Rehabilitation	73.3	4.0	6.7	1.3	75
Prophylactic procedures	95.6	0.0	3.3	0.0	274
Fractures	20.0	15.0	5.0	70.0	20
Internal injuries	0.0	0.0	0.0	100.0	1
Dislocation	0.0	0.0	0.0	100.0	2
Strains and sprains	92.4	4.8	0.8	1.3	709
Lacerations	95.3	1.2	1.4	1.9	2,202
Superficial injuries	96.9	1.0	0.6	1.3	685
Contusions	89.6	4.6	2.4	3.0	839
Adverse affects of industrial substances	90.4	1.2	1.4	6.8	644
Burns	97.5	0.5	0.7	0.7	408
Other accidents	89.7	4.6	0.0	3.4	87
All diagnoses	93.1	3.8	1.1	1.5	13,503

No diagnosis recorded for 35 contacts

(From McEwen et al. 1981)

TABLE 5.6

Proportions of adults and children taking different sorts of medicines
during a 24-hour and two-week period

Type of Medicine	ADULTS		CHILDREN	
	Taken in last 24 hrs	Taken in last 2 weeks	Taken in last 24 hrs	Taken in last 2 weeks
	%	%	%	%
Gargles or mouthwashes	2	5	-	-
Health salts	3	8	1	3
Indigestion remedies	5	14	2	3
Laxatives	4	9	1	3
Suppositories	-	1	-	-
Throat or cough medicines or sweets	6	13	4	12
Cold or congestion relievers	2	4	1	4
Asprin or other pain-killers	14	41	5	18
Sedatives, sleeping tablets, tranquilliers	8	10	1	2
Anti-depressives, stimulants, pep pills	1	1	-	-
Skin ointments, antiseptics	8	14	10	19
Eye drops, lotions, ointments	2	4	1	2
Embrocation or ointment to rub in	2	7	1	2
Inhalants, drops or things to sniff	3	4	1	2
Diarrhoea remedies	-	1	-	1
Corn pads, foot powders, creams or dressings	3	7	-	1
Tonics, rejuvenators	3	5	2	2
Slimming aids	1	1	-	-
Vitamin tablets	5	6	5	6
Medicinal foods	3	4	3	4
Surgical clothing, trusses, bandages, elastic stockings	6	8	1	3
Alcohol - for medicinal purposes*	2	4	-	-
Hormones (or contraceptives pills)*	3	4	-	-
Travel or other kind of sickness pills	-	1	-	-
Other	16	22	6	10
	1,412	1,412	519	519

* These were not included in the children's check list, contraceptive pills were
only asked about if the informant was a woman.

(From: Dunnell & Cartwright - 1972)

TABLE 5.7

Medicines and appliances, by percentage of all respondents who had used
them in the previous fourteen days, for all sources of prescription

Type of Medicine	Percentage of respondents (100% = 2,153)	No. of brands in each group	
Analgesics	38.1	22	(4.5%)
Other medicines and means	27.1	85	(17.5%)
Skin medicines	20.4	70	(14.4%)
Appliances	15.3	37	(7.6%)
Other and unspecified medicines	13.4	Unknown	
Lower-respiratory medicines	13.1	37	(7.6%)
Antacids	12.1	22	(4.5%)
Counter-irritants	10.8	34	(7.0%)
Tonics and vitamins	10.8	42	(8.6%)
Salts	10.7	9	(1.9%)
Laxatives and purgatives	9.1	24	(4.9%)
Medicines usually medically prescribed	6.3	27	(5.6%)
Upper-respiratory medicines	4.8	24	(4.9%)
Eye and ear medicines	4.2	16	(3.3%)
Sedatives	3.8	6	(1.2%)
Antibiotics and other anti-infective agents	3.2	12	(2.5%)
Heart, urinary, and kidney medicines	2.6	7	(1.4%)
Other gastro-intestinal medicines	1.5	12	(2.5%)
Total		486	(100.0%)

(From: Wadsworth, Butterfield & Blaney, 1971)

TABLE 5.8

Lifetime prevalence compared with present use ranked by
percentage reporting each

	Lifetime prevalence rank	Present Use (regular or occasional rank)
Asprin	1.5	1.0
Beer, Wine	1.5	2.0
Alcoholic spirits	3.0	3.0
Tobacco	4.0	4.0
Painkillers	5.0	10.0
Laxatives	6.0	6.5
Anxiety-control agents	6.0	5.0
Sleeping aids	7.0	8.0
Health and appearance aids	8.0	6.5
Stay-awakes	9.0	9.0
Anti-allergy	10.0	10.0
Birth control	11.0	12.5
Weight control	12.0	14.5
Amphetamines	13.0	14.5
Antidepressants	14.0	12.5
Marijuana	15.0	16.0
Proprietary remedies for "kicks"	16.0	17.0
Heroin, cocaine, etc.	17.0	20.5
Hallucinogens	18.0	18.5
Volatile intoxicants	19.0	20.5
Sex increasing preparations	20.0	18.5
Sex decreasing preparations	21.0	20.5

From: Blum, 1971

TABLE 5.9

Medicines suggested by doctors as being suitable for self-medication
and the percentage of the population taking such with or without
a doctor's prescription

Medicine	Percentage of doctors suggesting it	Percentage of population taking it	
		without prescription	without prescription
Asprin	50	17.9	0.9
Indigestion remedies	30	10.7	1.3
Cough remedies	27	3.4	1.6
Laxatives	27	6.2	2.7
Anaglesics	25	33.0	5.0

Sources: For medicines suggested, Market Investigations Ltd. (1966)
For percentage of population taking such medicine,
Wadsworth et. al., (1971)
For with/without prescription figures, OPCS (1973)

(From: Williamson & Danaher, 1978)

TABLE 5.10

General Practitioners' evaluation of self-treatments

Evaluation	Percentage of Treatments
Completely adequate	24
Partially adequate	51
Harmless	11
Potentially harmful	5
Doctor did not know what was in the remedy	9

Source: Danaher (1976)

(From: Williamson & Danaher, 1978)

NOTES

1.   Quoted in Massey RU. Educating for Change: The Next 25 Years. Connecticut Medicine 1976; 40: 713-717.

2.   Osler Sir W. Quoted in Malleson A. Need Your Doctor be so Useless? London: George Allen and Unwin, 1973, p.77.

3.   Webb S. & W. The State and the Doctor London: Longmans, 1910, p.230.

4.   Stimson GV. & Webb B. Going to See the Doctor London: Routledge and Kegan Paul, 1975.

5.   Tuckett D. An Introduction to Medical Sociology London: Tavistock, 1976.

6.   Robinson D. Patients Practitioners and Medical Care. Aspects of Medical Sociology London: Heinemann, 1973.

7.   Farmer M. The Family: The Social Structure of Modern Britain 2nd Edit. London: Longman, 1978.

8.   Adams BN. The American Family, a Sociological Interpretation Chicago: Markham Publishing, 1971.

9.   Pratt L. The Significance of the Family in Medication. Journal of Comparative Family Studies 1973; 4: 13-35.

10.   Editorial. Holistic Medicine. The New England Journal of Medicine 1979: 300: 312-313.

11.   Wadsworth MEJ., Butterfield WJH., Blamey R. Health and Sickness: The Choice of Treatment London: Tavistock, 1971.

12.   Logan WPD. and Brooke EM. The Survey of Sickness 1943 to 1952 General Register Office Studies on Medical and Population Studies, No 12. London: H.M.S.O. 1957.

13.   Bell JM. The Use of General Practitioners Services by Young Married Women in a New Town B. Phil Thesis, University of Dundee, 1977.

14.   Bell JM., Black I., McEwen J. and Pearson J. Patterns of Illness and Use of Services in a New Town: A Preliminary Report. Public Health 1979; 93: 333-343.

15.   Dunnell K. and Cartwright A. Medicine Takers, Prescribers and Hoarders London: Routledge and Kegan Paul, 1972.

16.   Department of Health, Education and Welfare. Acute Conditions, Incidence and Associated Disability New York: US Centre for Health Services, 1969.

17.   Hinkle L., Redmont R., Plummer N. and Wolfe HG. An Examination of the Relation between Symptoms, Disability and Serious Illness in Two Homogenous

Groups of Men and Women. American Journal of Public Health 1960; 50: 1327-1336.

18. Morrell DC. and Wale CJ. Symptoms Perceived and Recorded by Patients. Journal of the Royal College of General Practitioners 1976; 26: 398-403.

19. Alpert JL, Kosa J. and Haggerty RT. A Month of Illness and Health Care among Low-Income Families. Public Health Reports 1967; 82: No 8: 705-713.

20. Department of Health Education and Welfare. Chronic Conditions Causing Activity Limitation. Series 10 No 51: New York: US Centre for Health Statistics, 1969.

21. Fry J. A New Approach to Medicine Lancaster: M.T.P. Press, 1978. p.35.

22. Royal College of General Practitioners. Present State and Future Needs of General Practice 3rd edition. Reports from General Practice, No 16, London: Journal of the Royal College of General Practitioners 1973.

23. McEwen J., Pearson JCG. and Langham A. What Patients bring to Occupational Health Services Public Health 1981 95: 322-333.

24. Knapp DA. and Knapp DE. Decision Making and Self-Medication. American Journal of Hospital Pharmacy 1972; 29: 1004-1012.

25. Roney JG. and Nall ML. Medical Practice in a Community: An Exploratory Study Quoted in Pratt L. (reference 9), 1966.

26. Johnson and Johnson. Medicine Chest Survey Quoted in Pratt L. (reference 9), 1970.

27. Leach RH. and White PL. Use and Wastage of Prescribed Medicines in the Home. Journal of the Royal College of General Practitioners 1978; 28: 32-36.

28. Jeffreys M., Brotherston JHF. and Cartwright A. Consumption of Medicines on a Working Class Estate. British Journal of Preventive and Social Medicine 1960; 14: 64-70.

29. Hannay DR. The Symptom Iceberg. A Study of Community Health London: Routledge and Kegan Paul, 1979.

30. Kohn R. and White KL. (Eds.) Health Care. An International Study London: Oxford University Press, 1976.

31. Crooks J. and Christopher LJ. Use and Misuse of Home Medicines. In Anderson JAD. (Ed.) Self-Medication. Lancaster: M.T.P. Press, 1979.

32. Jones RVH. Self Medication in a Small Community. Journal of the Royal College of General

Practitioners 1976; 26: 410-413.
  33. Martindale. The Extra Pharmacopoea 27th edition. London: The Pharmaceutical Press, 1977.
  34. Eliott-Binns CP. An Analysis of Lay Medicine. Journal of the Royal College of General Practitioners 1973; 23: 255-264.
  35. Williamson JD. and Danaher K. Self-care in Health London: Croom Helm, 1978.
  36. Anderson JAD., Buck C., Danaher K. and Fry J. Users and Non-users of Physicians. Journal of the Royal College of General Practitioners 1977; 27: 155-159.
  37. Lader S. A Survey of the Incidence of Self-medication. Practitioner 1965; 94: 132-136.
  38. Festinger L. A Theory of Cognitive Dissonance London: Tavistock, 1962.
  39. Blum RH. Normal Drug Use. In Dreitzel HP. (Ed.) The Social Organisation of Health. Recent Sociology No 3. London: Collier MacMillan, 1971.
  40. Hassinger EW. and McNemara RL. The Families, Their Physicians, Their Health Behaviour in a Normal West Missouri County Quoted in Pratt L. (reference 9), 1960.
  41. Food and Drug Administration. A Study of Health Practices and Opinions U.S. Department of Health Education and Welfare, 1972.
  42. Roughmann KJ. and Haggerty RJ. The Diary as a Research Instrument in the Study of Health and Illness Behaviour. Medical Care 1972; 10: 143-163.
  43. Department of Health and Social Security. Eating for Health London: H.M.S.O., 1978.
  44. Stimson GN. Obeying Doctor's Orders: A View from the Other Side. Social Science and Medicine 1974; 8: 97-104.
  45. Garfield E. Patient Compliance: A Multi-faceted Problem with no Easy Solution. Current Contents 1982; 37: 5-13.
  46. Ley P. Communication in the Clinical Setting. British Journal of Orthodontics 1974; 1: 173-177.
  47. Porter AMW. Drug Defaulting in General Practice. British Medical Journal 1969; 1: 218-222.
  48. Parkin DM., Henney CR., Quirk J and Crooks J. Deviation from Prescribed Drug Treatment after Discharge from Hospital. British Medical Journal 1976; 2: 686-688.
  49. Linnett M. Prescribing Habits in General Practice. Proceedings of the Royal Society of Medicine 1968;1 61: 613-615.
  50. Manasse AP. Repeat Prescriptions in General Practice. Journal of the Royal College of

General Practitioners 1974; 24: 203-207.

51. Austin R. and Parish P. Prescriptions Written by Ancillary Staff. Journal of the Royal College of General Practitioners 1976; 26: Supplement 44-49.

52. Madeley J. Repeat Prescribing via the Receptionist in a Group Practice. Journal of the Royal College of General Practioners 1974; 24: 425-431.

53. Balint M., Hunt J., Joyce D., Marinker M. and Woodcock J. Treatment or Diagnosis London: Travistock, 1970.

54. Mapes R. Prescribing Practice and Drug Usage London: Croom Helm, 1980.

55. Jones DR. Errors on Doctors Prescriptons. Journal of the Royal College of General Practitioners 1978; 28: 543-545.

56. Chandler D. and Dugdale AE. What do Patients know about Antibiotics. Letter, Lancet 1976; 2: 422.

57. Fink JL. Self-medication. American Journal of Pharmacy 1976; 148: 90-96.

58. Stockley IH. Drug Interaction Alert. Aide-memoire on Interaction for Physicians and Pharmacists. Brackwell, Boehringer-Ingelheim, 1978.

59. Hart FD. Therapeutic poison pictures. World Medicine 1968; 4, No 3: 57-61.

60. Bodley Scott Sir R. (Ed.) Price's Textbook of the Practice of Medicine 12th edition. Oxford: Oxford University Press, 1978. p.271.

61. Davis SS. and Aslam M. Health Care needs of Asian Immigrants. Public Health 1979; 93: 274-284.

62. Ali AR., Smales ORC. and Aslam M. Surma and Lead Poisoning. British Medical Journal 1978; 2: 915-916.

63. Editorial. Liver Injury, Drugs, and Popular Poisons. British Medical Journal 1979; 1: 574-575.

64. Fryers GR. Products for Home Medication. In Anderson JAD. (Ed.) Self-Medication Lancaster: M.T.P. Press, 1979.

65. Cargill D. Self-treatment as an Alternative to the Rationing of Medical Care. Lancet 1967; 1: 1377-1378.

66. Charney E. Compliance and Prescribance. Marginal Comment. American Journal of Diseases of Childhood 1975; 129: 1009-1010.

67. Parish P. Medicines. A Guide for Everybody Harmondsworth: Penguin, 1976.

68. Golden R. Patient Delay in Seeking Cancer Diagnosis: Behavioural Aspects. Journal of Chronic

Diseases 1963; 16: 427-431.

    69.   Breckon W. The Physick in the Herbs. World Medicine 1977; 12 No 22: 44-49.

    70.   Office of Health Economics. Without Prescription. A Study of the Role of Self-Medication London: O.H.F., 1968.

    71.   Rea JN., Newhouse ML. and Halil T. Skin Diseases in Lambeth. British Journal of Preventive and Social Medicine 1976; 30: 107-114.

    72.   Ryan M. Self-diagnosis. British Medical Journal 1979; 2: 979-980.

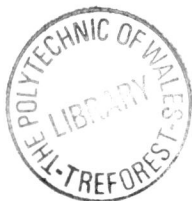

Chapter Six

PROFESSIONAL PRIMARY CARE:
IS THERE ROOM FOR PARTICIPATION?

"Self-reliance and social awareness are key factors
in human self-development. Community participation
in deciding on policies and in planning, implementing
and controlling development programmes is now a
widely accepted practice."(1) Although it was felt
that participation in planning and provision of
health services was in most aspects distinct from the
main concern of this review, it was considered that
it would be inappropriate not to refer to it and, in
particular, that the development of participation in
the provision of primary care services was of direct
relevance. Two aspects of the patients' role are
discussed: firstly, their role in the health centre
and secondly their role in the individual treatment
they receive from their general practitioner
(although some aspects of this are covered in other
chapters).

THE COMMUNITY HEALTH CENTRE

A discussion of the state of participation in health
centres cannot ignore the "Peckham Experiment" of the
1930's. (2) This began with a small group of lay
people, all under 30, who believed that health was a
factor of primary importance for human living.
Although they had no clear idea of what they meant by
'health', they sensed that its secret lay with the
infant and its early development. They therefore
distinguished their major areas of concern: that
parents should be sickness-free before the
conception of the child; that conceptions should be
wanted and that the parents should have comprehensive
knowledge and facilities to care for the child.
Families were offered a health service made up on the

structure of a Family Club, including general health checks and ancillary services for particular groups, such as babies.

The founding ideas also included an awareness of the futility of sending individuals back to the same poor environment responsible for the health problem and aimed to provide what it termed "instruments of health".

The concept was realised in the years 1935-1939 with the founding of the Pioneer Health Centre in Peckham. It re-opened in 1946 after the War, but thereafter faded with the introduction of the National Health Service. It is interesting to note that at the beginning of the 1980's a small group who have kept the concepts of the approach alive are attempting to set up a new experimental centre, using the same philosophical approach. Such a new centre, if it was established on the basis of a combination of the aims and enthusiasm of the original group and the advances and research that have come from both medical and social sciences during the intervening years, might provide the opportunity for an exciting development in primary health care and produce invaluable research material.

The notion of the community health centre has enjoyed a revival recently; Malleson (3) is one commentator who has brought to our attention the value of such schemes. He enumerates what he sees as the essential characteristics of a health centre:

> a building specifically designed to accommodate all the medical and social care facilities and staff needed to promote the individual and general good health of the people of the surrounding community. A health centre is particularly concerned with the prevention of disease and injury, and in providing necessary help for the sick and disabled within their own homes and neighbourhoods. A health centre offers care to the sick with the exception of those who require that twenty-four hour nursing and medical care that only a hospital can provide. A health centre shares with other centres a back-up hospital to which such sick patients are referred. A community and its centre together determine the policies of the centre and the nature and extent of the centre's work ...

He points out why he considers that health care based on health centres would probably work better:

1.   Health centres can prevent illness better.
2.   Health centres can more easily set realistic limits to the extent of care that they provide, both to the community at large and also to individuals.
3.   Health centres rationalize the present arrangements for providing social and medical care, and they make the provision of such care both more effective and less expensive.
4.   Health centres can help people to organize to help themselves.
5.   Health centres research into the needs of their communities and study the effectiveness of the services they render. They also provide a setting in which doctors and other professional helpers can be trained to provide useful care.

In addition to the curative functions of a health centre, there are opportunities for prevention and health promotion. This is now receiving more attention and the Royal College of General Practitioners (4) has introduced the term "anticipatory care", to imply this union of prevention with care and cure - 'prevention' including both the promotion of health and the prevention of disease.

Health centres provide the possibility for a variety of health professionals, who because of the diverse functions of a centre, visit it, to develop new working relationships. Hilton (5) notes, with particular reference to health education, the importance of providing suitable rooms and facilities in the planning of new health centres. Hubley (6) using the community development approach, which has resulted from Third World experience, suggests that the following dimensions will occur if this is adopted in Britain.
(a)   area-based and holistic
(b)   responding to felt need
(c)   development of self-help groups and volunteers
(d)   pressure and conflict leading to participation
(e)   ulitization of lay workers
(f)   action research.
He forsees that organizational factors and conflict between participation and the non-directive approach and professional training are likely to be barriers.

In situations where innovation is easier, such as new suburbs or new towns, multi-purpose centres involving education for young people and adults, day centres, clubs of various kinds and a full range of health services, are starting to develop. Sadly some of these fail to make use of the potential for co-operation and participation and the result is a collection of traditional and isolated services under a single roof.

It seems that if the concepts above were fully realised, health centres could be structures within the health service, but not isolated from other aspects of the community, through which individuals could begin to participate in the health care given and received in their community.

PATIENT PARTICIPATION GROUPS

Starting with a few enthusiastic general practitioners in the mid 1970's, the concept of patient participation in primary care has been translated into practice in a number of health centres and group practices throughout Britain. Dr Alistair Wilson who was one of the innovators has described the philosophy behind the present development. (7)

> There are many more patients than doctors and other health staff, whether we define a patient as someone who is ill or just someone who is registered with a general practitioner. The latter definition means the great majority of the population. The National Health Service belongs to them, not to the thousands of doctors nor even to the million people who work in the health service of this country. Thus it is strange, is it not, that so many have so little say in running or questioning the running of the NHS?
>
> The first reason, I think, that there should be participation by patients in the running of their general practitioner service is that it is a new form of democracy. Patients can elect their representatives to meet with and discuss the provision of general practitioner care with the doctors and other members of health staff.

At a conference held in Bristol (8) in 1977, there was an opportunity to assess the development of such groups, to explore their aims and activities and to consider the anxieties held by individuals and organizations. At this conference experiences were recounted and compared and it was found that the frequency of meetings varied between monthly and quarterly and that some operated 'social services' such as a Social Club for the mentally ill and baby-

and granny-minding and that topics covered in their numerous lectures and discussions (one practice has held 90 in 3½ years) included services for the elderly and children, self care, cervical cytology, screening cancer, abortion, patients' rights, drug abuse, sex problems, transport for hospitals visitors and yoga.

The declared aim of the Patients' Associations – also called Practice Associations and Community Participation groups – was to open a *channel of communication between patients and doctors.

The detailed functions of one such committee, as laid down in its constitution were: (9)

1. to participate with the doctors and other members of the health team in the running of the primary care service;
2. to consider complaints and improvements in the service;
3. to provide health education, lectures, and discussions to teach positive and preventive health, including the early signs and symptoms of disease;
4. to communicate the opinions of the patients to other bodies, such as the community health council, the health authority, local authorities, etc.;
5. to improve the levels of care available; and
6. to set up sub-committees to deal with various aspects of patients' needs.

At the conference (7) it was noted that the number of complaints resulting from the formation of groups, was not as great as many doctors had feared. One of the most positive aspects which had emerged was the education component with its accompanying exchange of views. There had been some hesitancy in taking up some of the social services offered, possibly, it was speculated, because of the stigma attached to attending as a client, which did not attach to the role of patient.

Most resistance to associations came from the doctors themselves. It was said that they:

> did not wish to be told how to run their practice, and some of them fear being seen as less than omnipotent. (In defence it was pointed out that many patients preferred their doctors to be somewhat removed and distant and would lose confidence if their G.P. tried to become an ordinary, approachable man-in-the-street).

This raises the interesting issue of what unforseen 'side-effects' there might be to the equalisation of doctor-patient relationships. The

conference raised too, the matter of reactions to the
Patients' Associations from the Community Health
Councils, some of whom were encouraging and even
initiating groups and others of whom were feeling
threatened. The latter: "... saw patients'
associations as unnecessary bodies duplicating
C.H.C.'s own efforts (and possibly usurping some of
their power?). They felt they were the appointed body
to deal with complaints and to liaise with F.P.C.,
D.M.T., A.H.A., etc."

The conference seems to have concluded on an
optimistic note, however, with a "... strong feeling
that patient associations rather than health centres
would be the most important thing to come out of the
health service in the next twenty years, and a great
deal of enthusiasm for a return of democracy."

Although there have been advances since that
conference, as is evident from the larger numbers of
groups in existence at the time of the Second
National Association of Patient Participation in
General Practice conference held in Oxford in 1979,
there was still at that time an expression of
uncertainty by the British Medical Association
Central Ethical Committee with particular reference
to the possibility of it being seen as 'advertising'
for a particular doctor or practice.

Patient groups have received the support of the
Royal College of General Practitioners (10) although
some general practitioners (11) have never heard of
such groups and were sceptical of the claims of
improved communications and feared possible trouble.
Such groups were seen mainly to exist in health
centres and not in single doctor practices or small
partnerships. Is it, as has been suggested (12) that
they are only necessary in larger practices and
health centres where there are problems of
communication?

To give an impression of the projects which are
taking place in this field, we have picked out a few
examples of such associations, both to describe what
is being done and to bring out some of the issues
which surround democratisation of primary care.

In Didcot, in England (13) a patient representative has been appointed to the health centre house
committee with the justification that there has been
a tendency for professionals to become superior and
dictatorial when insulated from direct confrontation
with patients' feelings regarding management
problems. The criteria felt to be particularly
important for such a person were the following:
1.   Detached from professions.

2.   Known to be receptive to complaints and problems about the health centre.
3.   Publicly known to be approachable.
4.   Could present problems to a professional committee in a sensible, detached and forceful manner with a sympathetic understanding of both sides of the health service.
5.   To be a patient registered at the health centre.
A woman who was the local Citizens' Advisory Bureau honorary organizer, already familiar with assessing the importance of public inquiries and complaints, in addition to complying with the above criteria, was appointed.

The following two examples also taking place within the National Health Service, illustrate the scope of such participation.

Of his Community Participation Group in Berinsfield, Oxford, Pritchard (14) reports that:

A two and a half year's experience of a community participation group has shown that this can have a valuable role in suggesting practicable improvements in a group practice ... The high attendance rates at the group's meetings testifies to the community's interest in primary health care services.

After initial reserve, it seemed ideas began to flow, giving both sides more understanding of others' problems. Health workers were reminded of the difficulties for single-parent families without cars and lay people gained insight into staffing problems during unsocial hours. Recommendations were implemented; for instance, there is now a chiropody service with transport, for the elderly; students are allowed in consultations only under certain conditions.

Dr Pritchard concludes his report with his hopes for the scheme:

If it succeeds, not only will it give us the opportunity to tailor our services to meet the needs of the community better, but it should also make health a matter of concern to the community, regardless of whether or not individual members are personally using our services.

When the Aberdare Health Centre opened in Glamorgan in July 1973 (9) it was decided straight away to have an elected patients' committee, on the grounds that:

> As doctors, we realise that the experience of six doctors is limited and so it seems sensible to us to tap the varied and unique experience and ideas of as many of the patients as possible. There is no suggestion of confrontation. The aim is quite simply co-operation between the patients and the health team, so that together they can improve the quality of the service. The service is a national one; it does not belong to the doctors - it belongs to the people. So it is natural that the people should take part in running it.

Because in Aberdare, 58% of the working people are manual workers, many in Social Class V, and because there was an awareness that the National Health Service worked on a 'come and get it' basis, resulting in the lower classes under-using available services, the Patients' Committee aimed to: "Encourage people to come early in their illness when so many lives can be saved and so much ameliorative treatment provided."

Like Dr Pritchard, Dr Wilson (7) stresses the two-way nature of communication. The staff have a chance to air their own problems but the net result has been to raise standards of care. Because of the opportunity to participate, the public is becoming more educated, more aware. And this in turn is having repercussions for the one-to-one relationship between doctor and patient.

> Another new concept in primary care is the involvement of the patient in making diagnosis; the open discussion by the doctor and the patient, meeting as two equal human beings with mutual trust and respect. Then there is also the discussion as to why a pill is to be given or not given, and if given what the possible side-effects may be. The patients are shown the consultants' reports and the doctor discusses and explains the contents. The patient is encouraged to ask questions - to say "Why doctor?" This is what is called open medicine. Clearly the greater the understanding of the patient the more useful his evidence will be and the more important his/her role in the diagnostic partnership becomes. I think medical care with the patient, not just for the patient, is the best kind of medicine. It is much better

also as a means of improving doctor/patient communication and relationships. If this kind of friendly discussion can be developed during a consultation, is it not sensible that it should also be continued by the health team meeting the representatives of the patients say on one evening each month?

Clearly the structure, the administration and the attitudes of the staff in a service and the quality of care cannot be separated, (which makes us realise the artificiality of the sub-headings of this chapter). Patients sharing in the running of the health service and patients sharing in their own treatment are interdependent - both breeding a sense of awareness and responsibility.

PATIENT PARTICIPATION IN CARE

Turning to the individual perspective and the task of encouraging participation from the individual patient's point of view, where does the doctor begin?

One basic barrier in the past has been the secrecy of medical records, of reasons for treatments, sometimes of prognosis and of the precise nature and effects of medication. Being kept in the dark has left the patient often bewildered and dependent.

A step forward would undoubtedly take place if patients were allowed full knowledge of their condition and treatment. This would also bring different worries to the patient, but then coping with realistic worries is part of the growing up of the patient. Participation aims to bring the patient from the state of childlike dependency, ignorance and obedience into a state of adulthood with its accompanying responsibility, power and autonomy.

Some doctors maintain that there are certain situations where the patient might be harmed by the truth, such as terminal illness, hereditary disorders and certain psychiatric conditions. There is no suggestion that unwelcome truths, or uncertainties during the early stages of investigation, should be thrust abruptly down an ill patient's throat or that patients who genuinely wish to remain ignorant must be told the details or the complications of their conditions. It is suggested that a more open approach taking the patient's desires and needs into account should be adopted.

Doctors are sometimes required to write

references, for example, in the case of adoption of a
child. If a doctor has written a comment detrimental
to the character of the patient, then it seems in
accordance with modern thinking that the patient
should have a right to know and contest such
judgement, when the consequences could be so far-
reaching.

The idea of patient held records has been
supported by a number of writers (15-16) who suggest
that it would improve patient knowledge and
compliance and increase communication between
various health professionals as well as between
doctor and patient. Indeed the use of 'co-operation
cards' has long been established in the care of
pregnant women. There are however other doctors who
are totally opposed to patient held records and the
British Medical Assocation considers that it would
lead to a deterioration in the doctor-patient
relationship. (17)

Hertz et al have reported on their attempt at
patient participation (18) using a system which
includes shared medical records. After six months
they found it had added minimally to the time
consumed and had been greeted with enthusiasm from
the patients. The basic components of this method
include such things as a health questionnaire,
immunization lists and progress notes, based on a
scheme devised originally by Weed. (19-20) In
addition, the patient participates in a one-page
'Health Care Plan' which consists of a form,
completed by the professional, in the presence of the
patient, along with a discussion on problems, their
solutions and continuing health maintenance. The
form is signed by both parties, each of whom keeps a
copy. The value of establishing an explicit contract,
now gaining some recognition among medical
practitioners, is well established in social work
techniques. (21)

This co-operative approach is echoed in a paper
by Dingwall (22) who describes his work, teaching
patients self-care in a new practice in Glenrothes, a
Scottish new town. It has already been recognized
that in some areas, for instance, diabetes, the
patient could and indeed must play an important part
in management of the disease. Dr Dingwall was
interested in applying this theory to commoner
conditions such as sickness and diarrhoea and also to
more serious illnesses, such as chronic bronchities.
He hoped to see a scheme: "Where the doctor and
patient work out a regime satisfactory to both,
resulting in better control of the conditions by the

patient, fewer episodes of crisis and better use of medical services."

Although there have been many accounts by patients suffering from almost the entire spectrum of disease, of the importance of participating in decision-making with regard to their care and their future, most of them have been individual accounts and there have been few studies which have sought to examine this critically. One exception to this is the field of terminal care where increasingly the value to patients and their family and friends of an open approach is being documented in a systematic manner. (23) The attitude of the patient is well summed up in the article entitled "Fighting Cancer - One Patient's Perspective". (24) The author describes the importance of the patient in decision-making as to the extent of surgery and the type and duration of drug therapy and the necessity for an holistic approach which recognizes that fighting cancer is more than excising a tumour and that patients must be equipped with a coping mechanism for improving the quality of their lives.

The desire by patients for more information about their conditions and the increasing demand for a reduction in medical secrecy may lead to a new open approach to care, and overcome the resistance of some of the professionals.

There seems to be two major ways of increasing the patient's participation in his or her own treatment. One is to have all records, letters, X-rays and so on, freely available to the patient; the other is to make the patient a partner in the decisions about treatment, with both doctor and patient agreeing on a certain course of action.

Although common sense would seem to encourage these approaches, such changes will have to be evaluated and be susceptible to criticism from both patients and professionals. What evidence is there that it would lead to improved health or quality of life? Perhaps raising the status, responsibility and self-respect of the patient is in itself, health-enhancing.

Before concluding this chapter, let us look briefly at three projects from around the world to see what other lessons there are to be learned.

Australia

Bates has described a scheme running in Australia, which began in 1974. (25) With the title of Consumer Health Involvement Project (CHIP), it established co-ordinators with the aim of working with people, learning how to bring about intelligent health consumers. They wanted to get to know the people in the area, gaining their interest and confidence, learning about their feelings and problems - through interviews and surveys in the shopping centre and at meetings with community groups.

CHIP has aimed to be flexible in firstly assessing and then meeting the needs of the community and aiding communication between its professionals and consumers. It has attempted to give people an understanding of the limitations of scientific medicine, increase awareness of health services and costs as well as their responsibilities and rights, the long-term goal being to involve consumers more closely in health care planning before they even need to use the services. It was hoped that there would be a gradual development of active educated consumers representing the public.

One of the points that CHIP brings home is a factor not yet discussed: the value of looking at health problems from the point of view of the public, finding out what they want, rather than what professionals think they want. Consulting the public could well avoid some costly errors and result in more commitment to, and better use of, the health services.

United States of America
Pearchik et al have devised a conceptual framework for participation and put it into practice in the Mon Valley area of Pennsylvania. (26) This system of participation works on a basis of committees to whom the Mon Valley Health and Welfare Council refers all requests, proposals and reports for their evaluation and recommendations.

One instance cited to illustrate the benefits of such lay involvement was the improvement in the methods of running blood banks. The old system was recognized by the professionals to be expensive and inefficient, but any action to ameliorate the situation was low down on their list of priorities. The lay participants, however, coming fresh to the system and being shocked by its inefficiency, initiated improvements which resulted in lowered costs for the hospitals and a more comprehensive service for the public.

Here, the value of the lay involvement was in looking at the problem with a new pair of eyes and not being so taken up in the day-to-day running of the health service that they could not see the long term benefits of - perhaps temporarily inconvenient -

changes in the system. Possibly too, there was a certain urgency of personal motivation. A health planner can say with some complacency that, say, 95% of the population has a supply of blood readily available, but to those who happen to be in the 5% that are not covered, the situation is unlikely to be seen as satisfactory and action more imperative.

Canada

Finally, we look at one instance where participation has led to considerable difficulties. Lay control was introduced at a medical clinic in Saskatchewan, in Canada, (27) but problems and conflicts ensued, with allegations from professionals of unchecked interference and lack of medical knowledge. This led to the resignation of all ten clinic physicians in 1974.

This brings home the point upon which a lot of issues of participation hinge - the balance between the aims, motives and rewards of those who have the special skills and provide the services and the needs of the patients and the community. Only by understanding these and by good communications between the two sides is there the likelihood of constructive changes.

CONCLUSION

Patient participation in the provision of primary care is established and growing as evidenced by the National Association of Patient Participation in General Practice. But is it to be welcomed without qualification? Should it be implemented everywhere?

There are many possible risks: that the people on the committee will not be representative, or that they will be overawed and dominated by the professionals, thus making the whole process mere lip service to participation. There are also dangers of an opposite nature: that the patients might prove too powerful and insist on professionals acting in accordance with their demands rather than relying on their own professional judgement. This might become a special risk if a committee came to be dominated by a particular pressure group.

In embarking upon the trend of patient participation, it is usual to make some assumptions and to begin with some axiomatic beliefs - such as, that patient participation can improve health - but whether or not the means are actually leading towards the desired end is a question which demands constant monitoring and evaluation. There could be a real risk that patient committees become just another layer of bureaucracy, slotted in, one level below the community health councils. It is interesting to note that several years after the establishment of community health councils there is still uncertainty and some confusion about their role and that although many councils have instituted exciting developments, there is great variation and the lessons learnt are not always applied elsewhere. (28)

The need to proceed in this type of participation seems to be justified from the results of surveys of public opinion about health services. Summarising the findings of such studies, some of which were specifically carried out for the Royal Commission on the National Health Service, (29) Klein (30) notes that there is overall satisfaction with the National Health Service, but that there are specific complaints and grumbles with younger people in general being more critical. The main sources of dissatisfaction fall into two categories: the organizational routine of hospitals and the personal attitudes of doctors among other members of staff. The problems of communication between doctor and patient both in hospital and the community stand out as the most important area of difficulty. While there are no quick solutions to some problems where the current financial constraints are likely to perpetuate some of the organizational limitations, it seems likely that these problems of communication which are seen to be so important, could be reduced or ameliorated if more participation by patients was encouraged, and that this would involve little or no cost.

One of the most pressing problems in the health services is that of scarce resources. (31) It seems that this may provide an impetus to look again at ways of improving primary care and of utilizing existing resources both professional and lay, to maximum effect. While it is important to overcome the problems of access to care (32) it is necessary to assess the quality of care as well as quantity. Locker and Dunt (33) agree that "studies of consumer opinion to the extent that they are taken into account in policy formulations, are an indirect form of consumer participation." There is need for a new comprehensive yet sensitive measure, a health indicator, which could be used to measure need for care, detect high risk groups and be used to assess outcome of care, both at the individual and group level. (34-35)

Van den Heuvel (36) reminds us that a conceptual clarification is needed in order to promote and apply the ideas implicit in the concept - 'the consumer involvement in health policy'. From a review of studies he concludes that:

- bureaucratic orientation in health care and the human rights movement promote the concept of the consumer in health care
- in the bureaucratic approach 'consumer' means control of costs-prices, outcome and efficiency, while in the human rights movement 'consumer' means self-control and participation
- the usefulness of the concept consumer in health care remains open to debate
- the idea of consumer participation is accepted in most health care institutions
- in most health care institutions a resistance exists to total consumer participation in policy making and evaluation of services, especially the quality of services
- the role of the consumer is a difficult one in the present relations within health care institutions, especially because of the differences in values and communication patterns
- the design of many studies dealing with consumers' satisfaction and evaluation have not the conditions to contribute to the involvement of consumers in health policy.

Progress along both conceptual and pragmatic paths will obviously continue and hopefully be linked. Currently individuals and groups who are committed to participation will continue to be most active, but will it remain an isolated phenomenon or will it become widespread?

Levin (37) who considers that the lay person should be recognized as the primary health care practitioner feels that an enhanced role of the patient can lead to an improved efficiency of the overall health care system and reduce the clearly evident public displeasure and thus, lessen the likelihood of conflict. This view is shared by Wilson (7) who states that: "the level of care particularly for the old, the young, the mentally ill and the disabled, have certainly been improved where there has been closer co-operation and joint activity of health staff and patients' groups." As is evident from the following phrase in the health education leaflet used in the health centre, Wilson has a vision of this new approach: "What is being attempted is to use the great untapped wealth of human understanding to fight the disease."

NOTES

1.   World Health Organization. Primary Health Care Geneva: W.H.O., 1978.
2.   Pearse IH. The Quality of Life. The Peckham Approach to Human Ethology Edinburgh: Scottish Academic Press Ltd., 1979.
3.   Malleson A. Need your Doctor be so Useless? London: George Allen and Unwin, 1973, p.195-196.
4.   Royal College of General Practitioners. Health and Prevention in Primary Care Report from General Practice 18. London: R.C.G.P., 1981.
5.   Hilton DD. Health Education in Relation to Health Centre Planning. Public Health 1981; 95: 90-96.
6.   Hubley J. Community Development and Health Education. Journal of the Institute of Health Education 1980; 18: 113-120.
7.   Wilson A. Patient Participation Will Mean a New Kind of Caring Service. Medical Sociology News 6, 1979; 2: 3-4.
8.   Report on Conference of Patients' Associations May 1977, Bristol. University of Nottingham, Department of Community Health.
9.   Wilson ATM. Patient Participation in a Primary Care Unit. British Medical Journal 1977; 1: 398.
10.   Norell JS. Patient Participation Groups. Journal of the Royal Society of Medicine 1980; 73: 697-698.
11.   Wood J. and Metcalfe DHH. Professional Attitudes to Patient Participation in Groups: An Exploratory Study. Journal of the Royal College of General Practitioners 1980; 30: 538-549.
12.   Editorial. Patient Participation: More Pipedream than Practice? British Medical Journal 1981; 282: 1413.
13.   Asbury JFP. Consumer Representation in Health Care Management. Lancet 1975. 1: 1187.
14.   Pritchard PMM. Community Participation in Primary Health Care. British Medical Journal 1975; 2: 583-584.
15.   Shenkin BN. and Warner DC. Giving the Patient his Medical Record. A Proprosal to Improve the System. New England Journal of Medicine 1973; 289: 688-692.
16.   Metcalfe DHH. Why Not Let the Patients Keep

their own Records? Journal of the Royal College of General Practitioners 1980; 30: 420.

17. First Word. Doctors are not Playing God by Keeping Notes Confidential. British Medical Association News Review 1980; May: 9-11.

18. Hertz CC., Bernstein JW. and Perloff TN. Patient Participation in the Problem-Oriented System. A Health Care Plan. Medical Care 1976; 14: 77-79.

19. Weed LL. Medical Records that Guide and Teach. New England Journal of Medicine 1968; 278: 593.

20. Weed LL. Medical Records. Medical Education and Patient Care Cleveland: The Press of Case Western Reserve University, 1969.

21. Rapoport L. In Roberts RW. and Nee RH. (Eds.) Theories of Social Casework Chicago: University of Chicago Press, 1970, p. 291.

22. Dingwall D. Patient Education in use of National Health Service Paper presented at 'Health Education and Primary Care Conference'. Dundee, 1975.

23. McIntosh J. Processes of Communication, Information Seeking and Control Associated with Cancer: A Selective Review of the Literature. Social Science and Medicine 1974; 8: 167-187.

24. Fiore N. Fighting Cancer - One Patient's Perspective. New England Journal of Medicine 1979; 300: 284-289.

25. Bates EM. Consumer Participation in the Health Services. International Journal of Health Education 1976; 19: 45-50.

26. Pearchik R., Ricci E. and Nelson B. Potential Contribution of Consumers to an Integrated Health Care System. Public Health Reports 1976; 91/1: 72-76.

27. Young KT. Lay-professional Conflict in a Canadian Community Health Centre: A Case Report. Medical Care 1975; 13/11: 897-904.

28. Levitt R. The People's Voice in the National Health Service London: Kings Fund, 1980.

29. Royal Commission on the National Health Service. Patients Attitudes to the Hospital Service Research Paper No 6, London: H.M.S.O., 1979.

30. Klein R. Public Opinion and the National Health Service. British Medical Journal 1979; 1: 1296-1297.

31. Office of Health Economics. Scarce Resources in Health Care London: Office of Health Economics, 1979.

32. Royal Commission on the National Health

Service. <u>Access to Primary Care</u> Research Paper No 6, London: H.M.S.O., 1979.

33.   Locker D. and Dunt D. Theoretical and Methodological Issues in Sociological Studies of Consumer Satisfaction with Medical Care. <u>Social Sciences and Medicine</u> 1978; 12: 283-292.

34.   McDowell I. and Martini CJM. Problems and New Directions in the Evaluation of Primary Care. <u>International Journal of Epidemiology</u> 1976; 5: 247-250.

35.   Hunt SM. and McEwen J. The Development of a Subjective Health Indicator. <u>Sociology of Health and Illness</u> 1980; 2: 231-245.

36.   Van den Heuvel WJA. The Role of the Consumer in Health Policy. <u>Social Sciences and Medicine</u> 1980; 14A: 423-426.

37.   Levin LS. The Lay Person as the Primary Health Care Practitioner. <u>Public Health Reports</u> 1976; 91: 206-210.

Chapter Seven

SELF-HELP ORGANIZATIONS

Appeals, in letters to the editor or on radio magazine programmes, from someone with a particular illness or problem, for others to join forces with them, to combat their common difficulties - to join in a self-help organization - are commonplace.

These problems are different from the everyday problems of life that come and go and are coped with. These usually are problems that continue and produce a significant effect on the way of life of an individual and related family members. Groups may be formed primarily from people with problems, they may include the relatives or there may be separate organizations for relatives of individuals with problems - such as the wives of alcoholics.

This sort of group is what usually springs to mind when people talk about self-help.

In this chapter we do not aim to supply a comprehensive list but rather to discuss, with examples, three facets of self-help groups:
1 an overall definition, through examination of their common characteristics
2. a typology of self-help groups, by pinpointing their differentiating characteristics
3. the internal organization and structure of self-help groups and how this reflects on their interaction with established professionals and organizations.

However, we once again come across the problem of definition - of what is meant by a self-help organization.

It is important here to differentiate between 'self-help groups' and 'voluntary organizations'. This distinction is discussed more fully in Chapter Twelve, but it is useful to note at this stage that self-help groups are run by, and composed of, the sufferers themselves whereas helpers in voluntary organizations are not usually also victims of the disease or problem. This distinction is not always absolute but provides a working definition.

In its review of community involvement, (1) the Volunteer Centre tackled the problem of definition by creating 4 categories:-

(a) services provided by or involving volunteers, voluntary groups and organizations within the sphere of social service, health, probation and after care, education, law, local government and the environment;
(b) the involvement of family, friends and neighbours in service provision;
(c) self-help and neighbourhood groups;
(d) community action and pressure group activity of all kinds.

This chapter will concern itself principally with the groups that fall into categories (c) and (d). Services provided by volunteers are normally more directly related to professionally provided services. These will be described later in the book in the context of changing professional roles.

COMMON CHARACTERISTICS

In the introductions to two of the main books describing self-help groups, (2,3) the authors comment on the meagreness of the research on self-help groups. A further American book by Riessman and Gartner (4) plus a number of articles often involving the same authors provide the basis of theoretical discussions and existing research.

Shipley, as editor of a Directory of Pressure Group and Representative Associations (5) makes the following general points:

The main requirement is that either category of organization is outward looking: the bodies concerned promote a cause or represent a defined group of people with the aim of bringing about changes favourable to that cause or group. Promotional and interest groups share in common the fact that they try to influence public opinion, directly through mass campaigns or indirectly through the media, and attempt also to shape the actions of government. They compete against each other in the allocation of resources and the determination of priorities, and on occasions appear at odds with the rest of society.

Self-help groups deal in many cases with problems which are serious, of a continuing nature and/or delicate, such as fatal or disfiguring illnesses, the death of a relative or uncontrollable phobias or obsessions. They have frequently developed as the result of a particular deficiency of care observed by a sufferer or by those who have cared for a sufferer of a problem or illness. Many of the problems are not regarded as strictly 'medical'. Stigmatized health conditions are an obvious focus. (6)

In short, the people who become members are often in a state of considerable distress about their condition. Such situations can lead people to feel very isolated. They feel that the medical personnel see a dozen patients like them everyday and have lost touch with the grief created anew for each patient at every diagnosis. And even those who are sympathetic are cut off from sufferers by the very fact that they are non-sufferers: they cannot know what it is like. This loneliness is brought to life by this illustration from Solzhenitsyn's "Cancer Ward":

> This harmonious, exemplary Rusanov family, their well-adjusted way of life and their immaculate apartment - in the space of a few days, all this had been cut off from him. It was now on the other side of his tumour. They were alive and would go on living, whatever happened to their father. However much they might worry, fuss or weep, the tumour was growing like a wall behind him and on his side of it, he was left alone. (7)

For these people behind Solzhenitsyn's wall - be it a tumour, a phobia or a bereavement - the existence of self-help groups may represent a sort of lifeline - a link, a bridge into companionship, a sense of belonging which the illness or problem has denied them. It offers a new reference group, a re-orientation from gazing on the blank wall of solitude to sharing in a society of like-minded people.

The literature of some self-help groups shows they are aware that their major function is to be an outstretched hand over that barrier: "The Compassionate Friends is an organization of bereaved parents who have been through their own heartbreak, loneliness and social isolation and can now offer help to others." (8) This enforced loneliness, this exclusion from normal social intercourse can be of a very practical nature, such as for those confined to a wheelchair, or it can be much more subtle.

This subtle exclusion is described in a book issued by the National Association for the Childless: (9)

> We do not know how to treat people who have not had or who do not intend to have children. In some sense they have offended against the implicit code governing human relationships, whether unintentionally or on purpose. They do not belong fully to the wider society.
>
> This is particularly hard for those people who do not choose to be childless, for they seem doubly deprived - of children and of a sense of belonging to the mainstream of society.

The considerable degree of distress, the isolation and its alleviation by the existence of self-help groups is exemplified in extracts from letters received from childless couples by the society:

> Sadly, I am one of the women you'll know so well ... I never stop counting days to my next period, hopeful fertile days, I sometimes drive myself crazy ... two days late and my personality changes, everyone is marvellous .. then the despair comes with the period. As soon as the worst is over, I'm planning next month, what I'll do and when, obsessive I know but I cannot help it.

> We thought about A.I.D. but everyone makes it out to be almost criminal.

> ... the part that hurts most of all is that we feel alone with our problems ... we have friends who have had children and drifted away.

> I was getting used to the idea of not having any children but this Christmas I received a card from someone saying have you any little ones yet and hurry up.

> When I see someone I know who has had a baby I feel deeply depressed. This one need seems to over-shadow all other things. I want to cry and cry and yet know no-one will understand me.

> We feel better writing this letter just to tell someone how sad we feel.

Our emotions are really taking a battering ...
how does one go about ceasing to try hard ... it
is difficult to be rational when deepdown I feel
obsessed by my own childlessness (and having an
abortion eight years ago doesn't help). I hope
and pray that you can offer us some small
comfort and advice. And thanks for existing. (9)

Two of the main features of self-help groups are
firstly that the problem or illness concerned be of
some gravity and secondly that the group has the
potential to help overcome some of the isolation, the
anxiety, uncertainty or frustration caused by that
problem. A further characteristic closely linked to
these is that those who have passed through the
crisis period and are back on an even keel, or have
learned to cope with the chronic problems of a
condition still feel sufficiently strongly about
their period of suffering that they are motivated to
help others in the same situation. This may be either
a feeling of banding together against a common enemy
or a sort of parental, protective attitude. Those
who have suffered in the past often have a desire to
turn a potentially negative experience into
something positive by building on their experience
and doing something constructive for others in the
same position. (10) They also feel that their
contribution is unique, that it constitutes an
expertise, one which is outside the scope of
professionals.

This means that, although all members have the
same problem, they are at different stages and this
lends optimism, some expectation of progress to those
in deepest difficulties.

Robinson and Henry (11) in describing how groups
accounted for their origins, found three main themes:
failure of existing services, recognition of the
value of mutual help and the role of the media. In
some cases, the disillusionment with existing
services and their failure to provide the necessary
help, advice, support and comfort, is associated with
an increasingly articulated anti-professionalism. In
certain instances, the failure of the services to
provide, may in fact be an inability rather than an
unwillingness to provide. It may be inappropriate, or
impossible for professional services to provide this
type of care. Some professionals may be just as
disillusioned as the patients.

Alcoholics Anonymous is perhaps the classical
example of recognizing the value of mutual help and
their approach has been taken over by other

organizations.

The media were often instrumental in bringing together those who felt alone with their problems, the severity of this problem often being not fully recognized by professionals or others until an individual account appears in the press, or on the radio or television. Other lonely sufferers "suddenly discovered" the extent of their shared problem and the desire for mutual support.

The Eraldin Action Group provides an example of a group seeking to help patients damaged by the side effects of practalol - a drug used in certain types of heart disease. This group has attempted to secure support from political and other sources for a campaign to recognize the clear links between the disabling condition and the drug and to pressurize for adequate compensation and the provision of appropriate services. In addition it draws attention to the whole problem of major drug tragedies such as thalidomide.

Does every chronic disease require its own group? Speaking at the inaugural meeting of the Motor Neurone Association, the founding member, who had been largely responsible for the organization, said: "only those suffering can really understand the distressing effects M.N.D. has upon the whole family. That is why an organization is needed." (12)

Since 'self-help' has come to refer to so many different activities there can be no easy or simple definition of what self-help really is. Nevertheless, the Self-Help Reporter, (13) the newsletter of the American Self-Help Clearing House, offered the following description which certainly highlights many of the familiar features of self-help groups:

> Their membership consists of those who share a
> common condition, situation, heritage, symptom,
> or experience. They are largely self-governing
> and self-regulating, emphasizing peer solidar-
> ity rather than hierarchial governance. As
> such, they prefer controls built upon consensus
> rather than coercion. They tend to disregard in
> their own organization the usual institutional
> distinctions between consumers, professionals
> and boards of directors, combining and
> exchanging such functions among each other.
> They advocate self-reliance and require equally
> intense commitment and responsibility to other
> members, actual or potential. They often
> provide an identifiable code of precepts,
> beliefs, and practices, that includes rules for

conducting group meetings, entrance require-
ments for new members, and techniques for
dealing with "backsliders". They minimise
referrals to professionals or agencies since,
in most cases, no appropriate day-to-day help
exists. Where it does, they tend to co-operate
with professionals. They generally offer a
face-to-face, or phone-to-phone fellowship
network that is usually available and
accessible without charge. Groups tend to be
self-supporting, occur mostly outside the aegis
of institutions or agencies, and thrive largely
on donations from members and friends rather
than government or foundation grants or fees
from the public.

Katz and Bender (14) use the following general
definition:

Self-help groups are voluntary, small group
structures for mutual aid and the accomplish-
ment of a special purpose. They are usually
founded by peers who have come together for
mutual assistance in satisfying a common need,
overcoming a common handicap or life disrupting
problem and bringing about desired social
and/or personal change. The initiators and
members of such groups perceive that their needs
are not or cannot be met by or through existing
social institutions. Self-help groups emphasize
face-to-face social interactions and the
assumption of personal responsibility by
members. They often provide material assistance
as well as emotional support; they are
frequently "cause" oriented, and promulgate an
ideology or values through which members may
attain an enhanced sense of personal identity.

Perhaps it is unrealistic to try and identify
the common features of such diverse organizations.
As a simple basis for working, recognizing that it is
limited, we suggest then that the defining
characteristics of a self-help group are thus: a
group created by those undergoing, or just emerging
from, an experience which has impaired their way of
life, to some extent, and which provides support for
themselves and for others in the same situation,
stands as a reference group for those isolated by the
crisis and offers some hope of improvement. (15)
The self-help movement is a social movement
which is change oriented - seeking to change its

members, or the public, or professionals or government or some combination of these. While generally it has been decided that individuals who are weak or oppressed band together defensively, as Katz and Bender point out, this viewpoint may be rather myopic: (16)

> It ignores the necessity so many people find to linking themselves to others for positive reasons, not just defensively, but as a way of claiming an identity, of asserting themselves and finding ways to live in a society that seems stale and un-nourishing to them.

Individuals come to realize that they have something special to offer - the "expertise of sufferers" - something which professionals and administrators cannot offer.

DIFFERENTIATING CHARACTERISTICS

If we were to provide a detailed and comprehensive categorisation of groups there really would be as many categories as there are groups. Categories cease to be very useful when they become too numerous. We will, however, refer to the main published works - some use the ideology of the group to produce the categories, while others use the structure or the problem that is being coped with.

We found the following simple classification used by Moore (17) in her book "Working For Free" useful. She distinguishes three types:
1.   Introspective, such as Alcoholics Anonymous or Compassionate Friends which provide comfort and 'therapy' for members.
2.   Pragmatic, such as the National Association for Gifted Children which provides courses for such children and advice for parents. Such groups tackle the problem themselves.
3.   Pressure Groups, such as the Patients Association or Disabled Income Group which pressurize official bodies.

Of course, some groups cover all three functions, either inadvertently or on purpose. For instance, although Alcoholics Anonymous specifically rejects political pressure as any part of its brief, by its very well-established existence, it does a public relations job for alcoholics. Also, the women in Italy who are setting up their own clinics (see chapter eight) may be thought to be acting pragmatically since, in the absence of a satisfactory state service, they are setting up their own. But they are also providing comfort and support for women and so belong to the 'introspective' category and, at the same time, undermining the authority of the weighty medical establishment by not submitting to their regime, and so are making a political point.

Other commentators have suggested different categories but we think these can be absorbed into this threefold typology.

Gartner and Riessman (18) propose four broad categories:

1. Groups engaged in rehabiliative work - helping the patients adjust to their new situation after initial medical care.
2. Groups concerned with behaviour modification in conditions such as alcoholism, drug addiction, over-eating and smoking.
3. Groups which provide primary care - usually where there is no 'cure' but where continued 'care' is required for a chronic condition.
4. Groups which encourage prevention or case finding. These are less developed but exist for hypertension and self-examination for breast cancer.

Katz and Bender (19) suggest five main groupings:

1. Groups that are primarily focussed on self-fulfillment or personal growth - "therapeutic" may also be used to describe them.
2. Groups that are primarily focussed on social advocacy - includes agitating and education directed at existing institutions, professionals, the public; confrontation, muckraking, and social crusading.
3. Groups whose primary focus is to create alter-native patterns for living. They may start new living and working alternatives.
4. "Outcast haven" or "rock-bottom" groups - a refuge for the desperate - usually involving total commitment in a living-in sheltered environment.
5. Mixed group - a residual category, where characteristics do not fit exactly.

Katz and Bender have also used another dimension - in which the main focus of the group dictates the category:

1. Inner-focussed groups, which are helpful to their members in material benefits, provide opportunities for personal grants, give emotional and social support, and offer many specific, concrete services.
2. Outer-focussed groups, where predominant interest is outside the immediate welfare of their

members, mainly devoted to changing legislation or social policy.

Gussow and Tracy (20) who concentrated on groups concerned with physical rather than addictive or mental health conditions, described two categories:

1. Type I groups which provide direct services to patients and relatives in the form of education, skills and encouragement - usually for conditions with no medical cure.

2. Type II groups which are more foundation-oriented promoting research, fund raising, public and professional education, and legislative and lobbying activities.

They describe how one organization, The Committee to Combat Huntingdon's Disease shifted from a Type I to a Type II organization early in its career.

Sagarin (21) differentiates between those groups which seek to make their members conform to society and those who seek to change the norms of society. Bean (22) postulates three kinds: 'crisis', 'permanent, fixed, stigmatized condition' and 'people trapped in a habit, addiction or self-destructive way of life'.

Whatever approach to categorization different authors choose, they all point out that they are not exclusive and that many groups - although emphasizing one approach, contain elements of other approaches.

It is not surprising that academics are groping for pigeon holes for self-help groups: there is always a desire to categorize and tabulate any new and expanding movement. But as mentioned earlier it is not really new. Demone (23) reminds us that such groups:

> are the fastest growing component of the human service industry. Nor is it surprising since man is a social animal who throughout his history has banded together for problem solving and survivial. Thus they are as old as men in one sense or a contemporary solution to complex problems in another.

We do not claim that Moore's three categories are definitive, but we hope that they will provide some framework for discussion - our aim being to illustrate the breadth and diversity of approach in the groups. One simple example of the differences is the use of the famous or relevant professionals. Some groups, more like the traditional voluntary organizations list prominent supporters, advisers and patrons, others make special mention of well known skilled professionals, others employ trained administrators. Many groups would see this as a denial of what they stand for and would limit their group to sufferers, family or involved friends.

Another feature which distinguishes groups is the degree to which the emphasis is on disseminating information. The main focus for some groups dealing, for example, with dietary conditions, skin problems and urinary infections may be to provide the patient or family with clear up-to-date information that will be of practical assistance. This may be a once off publication or a regular newsletter.

It is not possible nor appropriate to try to decide which is the best classification or to develop one that will encompass all others. We have found useful what Katz has said in a recent article. (24) He has:

> Formulated a number of differentiations that seem significantly to affect or even possibly to determine their structural properties.
> 1. The nature and intensity of the group's ideology.
> 2. Attitude towards professional help-givers and agencies.
> 3. The degree of identification with or rejection of the dominant society and its values.
> 4. The degree to which it employs such democratic practices as the rotation of leadership, and division of labour, as contrasted with centralization of power.

Katz concludes:

> The present need is not for more model building or classification schemes - a number of these exist. The need is rather for the much more arduous task of research - the accumulation of reliable data that will illumine proposed definitions, categories, and variable forms, and point to ways in which they need expansion or change.

One difficulty for both professionals and lay people with a problem is finding out what organizations exist and what sources of help and advice are available. An attempt to provide such information and to keep those in self-help movements informed has been undertaken by a self-help group. (25) In response to the rapid increase in the number of self-help groups and interest in them, the Self-Help Clearing House was formed in February 1977, at a meeting between SHARE Community Limited and two research workers who have been closely involved with a number of self-help groups. SHARE Community Limited is an action group offering self-help projects for disabled people. It was set up in September 1970 and achieved full charity status in November 1972. Since then, it has organized a number of self-help projects, with varying degrees of success.

The aim of the Clearing House was to provide a forum for exchanging ideas and practical information which could be helpful to those who are involved in some kind of self-help activity. The Clearing House accumulates information about self-help groups, their methods of working, their problems and their experiences, and shares this information with self-help groups and others who are interested in supporting its growth.

The Self Help Clearing House is, itself, a <u>self-help unit</u> and the people who work in it offer ideas and proposals on its strategy and management and bear responsibility for its efficiency.

> We want to provide an information exchange system between ourselves and other groups who can bring specialized skills and information, such as those groups who are active in health /welfare fields, industry and work-sharing schemes, communication media, housing cooperatives, community neighbourhood schemes, community health groups etc. We shall try to keep the system simple – but in anticipation of a growing response from a large number of groups covering numerous self-help activities, we already have contact with a self-help group in computer technology and intend using their service to assist our work.

This project is probably unique in that it was the first self-help information gathering and distribution unit in the U.K. to be established. The Self-Help Reporter (13) is the equivalent American publication. In Britain the Sunday Times Newspaper and the Kings Fund have both produced national directories of self-help groups.

WHAT MEMBERS GET AND GIVE

What individuals may get depend on their problem and their need. Some groups define their area of concern very narrowly, such as the Mastectomy Association who are concerned with the practical aspects of getting, wearing and living with a prosthesis. Contact is limited, and if there appears to be continuing or wider problems, the woman will be encouraged to seek help from some other source. Other organizations aim to provide much more comprehensively for an individual, and probably the family with the problem. Here, perhaps the greatest benefit is that of belonging, of not always being different from those around, of sharing with others who have the same or a similar problem. They are part of a structure – helping and giving to the organization, as well as receiving. There is opportunity for meaningful participation and making decisions, instead of always having someone else to make the decisions.

There is the opportunity to share information and problems and perhaps express secret fears which would be impossible in a less supportive environment – such as fear of battering a child. There are new friendships which will accept the individual for what he or she is, although frequently this may mean openly admitting to a problem, such as alcohol, instead of denying it. This is usually accompanied by admitting the need for help and wanting such help.

The provision of practical, yet authoritative help and advice on matters such as diet, exercise, shopping, special tools, etc., is a most valuable feature of organizations related to certain specific diseases such as diabetes, coeliac disease and phenylketonuria.

Individuals may gain from what they give to an organization – in participating in running it, raising money – either for support or research (this is more often a characteristic of the voluntary organization). The individual may be able to use pre-existing skills in providing leaflets, posters, driving minibuses, etc.

In all this there is a sense of belonging, of feeling that there is the possibility of improving matters and achieving some action. The individual has a reference group and frequently there is considerable improvement in self-esteem. There is a continuity of care that cannot be provided by any other approach.

In addition to the formal meetings, there is the importance of informal social contact: doing normal

things with new friends, but in an atmosphere where
problems are recongnized. The alcoholic, for
example, will not constantly be pressed to take a
drink, as occurs in normal social gatherings.

Such groups do not provide help or an acceptable
environment for all people with particular problems.
Some never contact them, others use them for the
practical help, but not the social interchange,
others try them briefly and find them unacceptable.
It would be surprising if this was not so.

ORGANIZATION AND INTERACTION WITH THE ESTABLISHMENT

> Say you decide you want to start a kind of self-
> help pressure group, what do you do?
> Once you have at least a few fellow
> supporters, you should call a general - public
> meeting.
> ... The next step is to have a steering
> committee appointed from the meeting ... whose
> job is to draft a constitution for the
> organization.
> ... experience has shown that organized
> groups get more done than unorganized groups.
> The Executive Committee elects its
> officers; usually a Chairman, Vice-Chairman,
> Secretary and Treasurer and perhaps a Publicity
> Officer ...
> ... Now you are organized, the action can
> start. (26)

Is all this sad proof of Weber's doctrine of
"the routinisation of charisma" which states that
spontaneous commitment to a cause tends to be
corrupted by the tendency of all organizations to
become 'ends in themselves'? (27) Or is it a
heartening illustration of how people are arming
themselves through organization against their
enforced powerlessness in many spheres?

Elsewhere we discuss the issues of participation and democracy in the professional sphere,
making the point that we cannot expect greater
equality, openness and mutual trust in professional-
patient relationships, if professionals themselves
cling on to the rigidly hierarchial relationships
which exist in the medical sphere.

Analogous to this is the issue we are putting
forward now - whether self-help groups can hope to
change anything if they are going to ape the customs
and organizational methods of the very institutions

which have failed them? Should self-help groups
'organize themselves' as Moore suggests? (26)
  Let us consider another viewpoint:

> Building an organization is not merely futile
> but dangerous: during those brief periods in
> which people are roused to indignation, when
> they are prepared to defy the authorities to
> whom they ordinarily defer ... those who call
> themselves leaders do not usually escalate the
> momentum of peoples' protests. They do not
> because they are pre-occupied with trying to
> build and sustain embryonic formal organi-
> zations in the sure conviction that these
> organizations will enlarge and become powerful.
>   ... virtually all who have had anything to
> do with the modern labour and socialist
> movements (except the anarchists) have hithero
> taken it for granted that the way to the future,
> whatever it might be, led through organization
> ...
>   ... that this must be the case seemed so
> evident and so clearly proved in practice that
> the belief itself was hardly ever investigated
> seriously.
>   ... radical movements which were not
> getting anywhere tended to substitute their
> organizational growth for real achievement and
> conversely that the concentration on the
> organization and its activities as such made
> them into participants in the system, led them
> to miss - or even worse to dismiss - various
> opportunities for struggle and produced various
> kinds of bureaucratic and digarchic ossific-
> ation. (28)

When applied to the field of self-help in
health, these two commentaries pose many questions,
which cannot be answered here, for they need further
empirical studies, but they raise important issues.
Do, or should, some self-help groups represent a
challenge to the medical establishment? If so, is
this best done by adopting the organizational
patterns of the establishment or by embodying
alternative methods and values? And indeed, if self-
help groups do not embody alternative methods and
values, are they fated inevitably to become like the
very organizations which provoked their discontent?
What imprint have these numerous self-help groups had
on our mode of living, both in the way we care for
ourselves and in the way we conduct treatment of

illness?

Dismayed by the degree of central control, Ward (29) sees self-help groups as hopeful signs and believes they have resulted from: "a consciousness that the machinery of central and local government exploit the impotence of the poor and are unresponsive to those who are unable to exert effective pressures for themselves."

And although governments have espoused self-help, seeing it as a chance of spreading departmental budgets further, Ward concludes gloomily: "you would have to look long and deep to find the slightest dent in the power structure".

Although he was referring to the total spectrum of self-help his comments can be applied to self-help in health.

Perhaps this is too pessimistic, but it does lend some perspective to the eagerly optimistic picture painted by some commentators. There is need for constant appraisal and readjustment. But although we admit that self-help organizations are not a panacea for the alienation and powerlessness often experienced by patients at the receiving end of health care they do represent a recognition of the need for a change in direction, in our methods of care, and for many people, very genuine solutions. The organizations vary enormously in their characteristics and aims but there is no doubt that they have not only made a considerable contribution to the quality of many lives but also their very existence and success in gaining support will gradually affect many other areas of society.

There are three main arguments against self-help groups. Firstly, that by relieving pressure on the official services and society they may discourage formal provison of such care - especially in the field of preventive services or already disadvan-taged areas, such as mental health. Secondly, there is a concern that groups may encourage "ghettoiz-ation", that people with a particular problem will be increasingly separated from, rather than integrated into, society. Thirdly, and this is related to the second charge, there is a fear that they will encourage dependency and indeed might further encourage the medicalization of human life.

While it must be admitted that in certain circumstances these fears might be realized, from reading the aims, objectives and activities of the many groups which communicated with us, it seems that these are unlikley to be serious problems. Katz (24,30) has argued convincingly against them all. He knows that people are always dependent on someone in one degree or another. The real question is the nature of that dependency. Is it self-chosen and does it reinforce the strengths of both parties involved? This kind of dependency is not in and of itself undesirable. The majority of care provided is social, educational and supportive rather than indirect in the strict sense.

Perhaps, instead of continuing to examine the groups, greater emphasis should be laid on looking at the relationship between existing organizations and professions and the various groups - to assess what can be learnt from their groups and what together will provide the best care for those in need. (31)

In conclusion, it is useful to remind ourselves of the positive contribution that is made by these groups to people who would otherwise have little encouragement and would not come to recognize their own potential.

> It may seem overdramatic to refer to the few hundred thousand, usually small and weak, self-help groups as necessary to the survival of their members. In a purely material sense, they may not be; their members would not die of hunger, exposure or disease in the absence of these supports. But to ensure an acceptable quality of life, humans need to recognize themselves and to be recognized by the society around them in all dimensions of their humanity. Survival in the modern world means more than having one's purely physical needs met; people must discover and be accepted for what they are. They need to live, to be valued, to experience, to give, to share with others, to transcend the boundaries of their own egos - to give and take in social communion. Many must fight for a place in the world, to reshape a society that cannot see their value.
>
> To us, that is why self-help groups have come into being; that is what they strive for; and that is why their importance can scarcely be measured by numbers, power or influence. (32)

The title of Katz and Bender's book on self-help groups in the Modern World "The Strength In Us" could not be more apt.

NOTES

1. Leat D. <u>Research   into   Community</u>

Involvement 1974-1977 Berkhamsted: The Volunteer Centre, 1977, p.3.

2. Katz AH. and Bender EI. The Strength in Us. Self-help Groups in the Modern World New York: New Viewpoints, 1976.

3. Robinson D. and Henry S. Self-help and Health. Mutual Aid for Modern Problems London: Martin Robertson, 1977.

4. Riessman F. and Gartner A. Help: A Working Guide to Self-help Groups London: New Viewpoints Croom Helm, 1980.

5. Shipley P. (Ed.) Directory of Pressure Groups and Representative Associations Epping: Basker, 1979.

6. Albon J. Dwarfism and Social Identity: Self-help Group Participation. Social Science and Medicine 1981; 15B: 25-30.

7. Solzhenitsyn A. Cancer Ward Harmondsworth: Penguin, 1971.

8. Compassionate Friends. No Death so Sad Leaflet from National Secretary: Mrs Joan Wills, 50 Woodwaye, Watford, Hertfordshire, WD1 4NW. (undated).

9. Houghton P. and Houghton D. Unfocussed Grief Birmingham: Birmingham Settlement, 1977, p.6 and pp. 47-49.

10. Finlayson A. and McEwen J. Coronary Heart Diseases and Patterns of Living London: Croom Helm, 1977.

11. Robinson D. and Henry S. Opus cit. 1977, p.12.

12. Southend - Journal of the South Nottingham Health District 1979; 5: No 34, Association formed by patients.

13. Self-help Reporter Published by National Self-Help Clearing House, New York.

14. Katz AH. and Bender EI. Opus cit., 1976, p.9.

15. Katz AH. and Bender EI. Opus cit., 1976, p.26-28.

16. Katz AH. and Bender EI. Opus cit., 1976, p.56.

17. Moore S. Working for Free London: Pan Books, 1977.

18. Riessman F. and Gartner A. Self-help Models and Consumer Intensive Health Practice. American Journal of Public Health 1976; 66: 783-786.

19. Katz AH. and Bender EI. Opus cit., 1976, p.36-41.

20. Gussow Z. and Tracy GS. The Role of Self-help Clubs in Adaptation to Chronic Illness. Social

Science and Medicine 1976; 10: 407-414.

21.   Sagarin E. Odd Man In: Societies of Deviants in America Chicago: Quadrangle Books, 1969, p.21.

22.   Bean M. Alcoholics Anonymous New York: Psychiatric Annals Reprint, 1978, p.38.

23.   Demone AW. Jnr., Introduction to Directory of Mutual Help Organizations in Massachusetts (4th edition) Blue Cross and Blue Shields, 1974.

24.   Katz AH. Self-help Health Groups: Some Clarifications. Social Science and Medicine 1979; 13A: 491-494.

25.   Share Community Limited. Self-help Spotlight London: Share Community Limited (ed.)

26.   Moore S. Opus cit., 1977, p.170-173.

27.   Weber M. The Routinisation of Charisma in Social Change, Etzioni A. and Etzioni E. (Eds.) 1964. Basic Books Inc. New York & London.

28.   Hobsbawm EJ. The Left and the Crisis of Organization. New Society 1978; 44: No 810, 63-66.

29.   Ward C. Self-help Socialism. New Society 1978; 44: No 811, 140-141.

30.   Katz AH. Quoted in Briggs HC. Conference on Self-help and Health: A Report. New Human Sciences Institute. New York: Queen's College, C.U.N.Y., 1976. p.11.

31.   Jones P. The Emergence of Self-help Groups. The Health Education Journal 1980; 39: 84-87.

32.   Katz AH. and Bender EI. Opus cit., 1976, p.3.

Chapter Eight

THE WOMEN'S HEALTH MOVEMENT

"When the social history of the 20th Century is
written, the 1970's will be seen as a time when women
began to seek a greater say in the management of
fertility, pregnancy and childbirth ..." (1)
        This phenomenon, noted here in the Lancet, has
come to be known as the women's health movement.

A NEW APPROACH

The concept of women's health as a discrete, homogen-
eous, political phenomenon originated in the U.S.A.
in the late 1960's. The women's health movement
created a perspective which differed from the
traditional approach to health problems in the
following ways:-
1.   the patient population was defined in terms of
sex rather than disease;
2.   improved treatment regimes were seen as being
necessarily preceded by a redistribution of power and
not attainable within the present system of health
care;
3.   the impetus to change in health care practices
was perceived as being in the hands of lay people
(both in terms of administering treatment directly
and in being responsible for pressurising for changes
in professional practices) rather than being left
entirely up to initiatives by health professionals
such as doctors, nurses, planners and researchers;
4.   deficiencies were perceived as arising from the
conflict of interests between patients as a group and
doctors as a group.
        This chapter will look at how and why the
women's health movement arose, its characteristics
and philosophy and what it hopes to achieve.

124

ORIGINS

The beginning of the women's health movement in the
United States of America can be seen as the fusion of
two social movements: health consumerism and the
women's liberation movement.

Health Consumerism

In the 1960's the consumer movement developed on both
sides of the Atlantic in many spheres of life,
including health. Doctors became the producers of
health care and patients, the consumers. These
consumers were conscious of their right to expect a
good quality product. Consumerism in health was not,
however, a new phenomenon in the United States of
America. The first such movement occured in the
1830's and 40's. What historians later called the
"popular health movement" brought together both
working class radicals and feminists who were seeking
a restructuring of health care. 'Doctor craft' was
denounced as elitist and un-American. This movement
declined however, to re-emerge in the 1950's as a
call for a rationalised health service - securely
financed and equitably distributed (2). The 1960's
saw a shift in emphasis from the demand for better
professional services to an interest in lay
participation. The era of protest movements brought
with it a mistrust of authority and the notion of
community control. Urban black groups became
dissatisfied because they perceived their health
services to be dominated by distant academically-
oriented medical centres. They started to campaign
not only for free health care but also for health
institutions to be controlled by local people.

This step towards community-controlled services
was also taken by the abortion campaigners whose
activities gave rise to the women's health movement.
They moved from seeking changes in the abortion laws
to seeking ways of they, themselves, controlling
health services for women.

The Women's Liberation Movement

The women's liberation movement is seen traditionally as having its roots in the 19th century
emancipation movements and subsequent suffragette
campaigns. Its decline after World War I was
succeeded by a lull in visible activity and
ultimately the movement's re-emergence in the
1960's. Its philosophy and aims have been charted

elsewhere (3) but it can be said here briefly that women in the 1960's were expressing increasing dissatisfaction with their roles at home, at work, in the legal system, financially and in many other spheres of life. Where they had attributed such dissatisfaction in the past to individual deficiencies, they began to look critically at the nature of the traditional female role. (4) They sought solutions, no longer in terms of adapting individuals to the social structure, but in changing the social structures. This new perspective required three preconditions, according to Oakley:

> 1. a widespread discordance between subject-ive reality and social norm;
> 2. the opportunity for its victims to compare experience;
> 3. some feeling of personal or collective efficacy in bringing about the kind of social change that can transform the material and psychological basis of oppression. (5)

GYNAECOLOGICAL SELF-HELP

The issue of abortion was one around which the early American liberationists rallied. They found, however, that the liberalising of abortion laws in the late 1960's was not the panacea they had hoped for. Availability varied from place to place. Dissatisfaction was expressed with the treatment, both in technical and personal terms. And so following the 'community control' trend, the campaigners addressed themselves to the question of how women might have some influence on the abortion service. In the words of Marieskind and Ehrenreich, both editors of women's health journals in the 1970's:-

> Abortion activists who had lobbied, counseled, or done illegal abortions before the liberal-isation of abortion laws now found themselves pitted against a medical system which effectively had the legal sanction to determine all the aspects of delivery of abortion care. (5)

At this stage two women came to prominence who were to be seen as founders of the American women's health movement. Carol Downer and Lorraine Rothman met with other women in Los Angeles to discuss the possibility of lay women having some control over the abortion service. This led to the undertaking of a programme of biological and medical education for themselves. This in turn led to broader philosophical and political discussions and the idea of gynaecological self-help.

Gynaecological self-help involved mutual education by sharing knowledge and experiences. It involved both self-examination and the gathering and reassessment of medical information. It was also concerned with the development of a political stance whereby health issues became the central area for some factions of the women's movement. Hornstein, Downer and Farber who were all directors of the Feminist Women's Health Centre in Los Angeles wrote:

> As we have grown, the self-help clinic has remained the backbone of our movement. It is our everyday experiences, examination of our own bodies and our lives that have led us to the political conclusions we have. Women see clearly that a prerequisite for their participation in social change is gaining control of their own reproduction. (7)

The concept of gynaecological self-help was presented by Downer and Rothman to the national convention of the National Organisation of Women (N.O.W.) in September 1971. This provoked invitations from other groups who wanted to learn self-help principles and techniques. Downer and Rothman undertook a six-week journey across the United States of America during which they taught women's groups, these groups contributing to the financing of each stage of the trip. They precipitated the setting up of 1,200 self-help groups and 50 feminist clinics.

In the summer of 1972, they acquired premises in Los Angeles which became the first "Feminist Women's Health Centre". In September of that year the centre was raided by the police who seized items and charged some women with practising medicine without a licence. One woman, Colleen Wilson, pleaded guilty to fitting a diaphragm and was find $250. The other, Carol Downer, who was alleged to have helped a woman diagnose and treat a vaginal infection, was acquitted, after two months of legal proceedings and $20,000 expenditure on legal fees.

The seventies saw women health activists elsewhere finding themselves in confrontation with the law. In 1979 Spanish police baton-charged a sit-in protest staged to express solidarity with women being tried on charges of illegal abortion. (8)

In 1977 a group of women in Berlin organised a lecture and demonstration about self-help and self-examination. A complaint to the mayor from a local representative of the Christian Democratic Party resulted in a vicious attack in the press and a demand for prosecution, on the grounds that the lecture was an invitation to lesbian love and could corrupt younger women. The prosecution was not taken up as no-one was named but the group was turned out of the adult education centre and so, writes Angela Phillips, reporting on the incident, "... they join a long line of women who have suffered 'Witch-hunts' because of their desire to understand and better control their own bodies." (9)

Women in China who refused compulsory abortion in 1981 found their electricity cut off and front doors sealed. If they fled, their husbands were imprisoned and many who refused were abducted and dispatched to hospital in pig baskets. (10) Women who tried to protect the pregnant women were officially dubbed 'sorceresses'! (11)

Indeed the use of the terms 'sorceress' and 'witch', usually intended perjoratively, has been taken up with pride by the women's health movement. A telegram in support of the American Women prosecuted for running a feminist clinic, from a well-known activist and writer Robin Morgan ran: "If they think they can burn witches and midwives again, they will be taught a bitter lesson STOP We must fight this first wave of a campaign to destroy feminist self-help medicine." (12)

Two writers who were early documenters of the women's health movement, Ehrenreich and English, have traced the movement back to the period of witch-hunts, pointing out that many of the 'witches' were in fact midwives who were condemned by the Church for administering herbal remedies to women in pregnancy and childbirth. (13)

These commentators have also charted some of the history of gynaecological surgery and describe a period in the 19th century when husbands took their wives to the doctor to be cured of such diseases as "troublesomeness, eating like a ploughman, masturbation, simple cussedness", by removal of the ovaries. (14) Indeed, as recently as 1982, a Harley Street doctor was performing an operation, described by the Royal College of Obstetricians and Gynaecologists as "barbaric, futile and illogical". The reasons given for the operation, surgical removal of the clitoris, were infertility, having had a previous caesarean section and "suffering depression and all that". (15)

Other instances of some of today's practices may appear to demonstrate little change. An International Conference on Women's Health in 1977 described some:

"... barbarous practices in some European hospitals such as: tying the hands of a woman in labour behind her head, administering general anaesthetic just as the baby is crowning (this is after the most painful stage of labour just before the most rewarding moment when the baby emerges). One practice witnessed was that of holding a women's legs together to prevent the baby emerging until the presiding doctor appeared - this was described as a 'method of torture which would make Amnesty International turn green'. (9)

Reports such as these, conferences, public debates, media coverage and a growth in feminist health literature have given rise to an ideology which focusses on the necessity for women to control their own fertility. Expressing this in the early days of the American movement, Tangri wrote:-

An accepted ethical principal forbids violating the bodily integrity of one person to secure the survival of another without the donor's consent. We would not consider it ethical to require a person to make his or her body available for organ transplants, experiments, or blood donations. Yet in the case of fertility, because continuation of the species requires that some women be fertile some of the time, all women are made to the social, legal, and political regulation of their reproductive capacity by others, mostly male.

Bearing children involves some or all of the following costs: invasion of the woman's body by the fetus; nine months of pregnancy; a period of restricted freedom while caring for the infant; risk of death, pain, disfigurement, major surgery (Caesarean) and permanent or temporary disabilities such as job discrimination against pregnant women and mothers. None of these costs are borne by men, and none should be imposed unwillingly on anyone. (16)

The wider women's movement has campaigned on many major issues: employment, violence, education, etc. There is however a substantial faction, the women's health movement, which regards the control of health care as central to the full emancipation of women.

The medical system is strategic for women's liberation. It is the guardian of reproductive technology - birth control, abortion and the means the means of safe childbirth. It holds the promise of freedom from hundreds of unspoken fears and complaints that have handicapped women throughout history. When we demand control over our own bodies, we are making that demand above all to the medical system. It is the keeper of the keys. (17)

It is evident that the women's health movement is an avowedly political movement, in which the feminist ideology of the wider women's movement is axiomatic.

AIMS OF THE MOVEMENT

In their book on self-care in health, Levin et al (18) note that "catching a social phenomenon in motion is a hazardous task". This is particularly true of the women's movement which tends to perceive as 'male', and therefore eschew the traditional structures of groups, such as committees and officials. There is no manifesto where the composite aims of all branches of the loosely-knit women's health movement are set out. The following are distilled from literature of the 1970's and early 1980's.

1. Demedicalisation

The women's health movement aims to remove some aspects of women's lives out of the medical sphere for two main reasons: (a) that some conditions are improperly defined as pathological. This is largely a reaction against the school of thought which attributes psychiatric disorders to women who are, for instance, pregnant, (19) childless, (20) failed contraceptive users (21) or intending to have an abortion (22). The movement argues that women in such conditions are making a normal response to a life crises (23). (b) That some conditions, whilst

130

properly defined as pathological, are not amenable to conventional medical treatment, and are, it is suggested, more effectively treated by homely and lay remedies such as dietary or life-style changes.

2. Redefinition of Roles in Medical Practice

Where medical intervention is necessary, the movement aims not to lobby for more of the present services but for a different type of service. In the feminist clinics, for instance, there is a doctor, but a great deal of the patient's contact is with lay women. The doctor's role is confined to specifically medical tasks such as prescribing drugs and performing abortions. The lay women, besides administering the clinics and providing counselling, encourage the patient to participate in her own treatment by, for instance, helping to interpret laboratory tests and teaching her how to examine herself and make early diagnoses. The emphasis is on the patient making as full a participation as possible and on the non-medical tasks often involved in medical practice being taken on by lay women.

An Italian clinic run on these lines by CRAC (Rome Committee for Abortion and Contraception) was described in 1977. Before consultations began women were invited to a collective discussion where those women who had attended before were asked to criticise their previous visit – what they disliked (if anything), how they would like this visit to be conducted, and whether they mind being examined collectively. It was reported that, on this last, there is no pressure: those who wish, can be seen separately, but most choose to go in groups of three. Usual consultations, therefore take the form of three women, two group members and the doctors.

In the words of one of the members: 'we ask the doctors to carry out their examination as <u>we</u> want them to, not as they are used to. We stay in here because we are paramedics, and want to learn as much as we can about health care. We also want the women to learn – about themselves and each other'. (9)

3. Promotion of Patient's Perspective

Many self-help groups and much self-help literature, arises out of a lack of congruence of views between doctor and patient on the importance of particular conditions, such as cystitis. (24) Because the doctor's training is primarily scientifically rather than socially oriented, the importance of an illness tends, for doctors, to be related to "the difficulty of its diagnosis or the complexity of its treatment rather than its effect on the patient's life". (25) The women's health movement - and indeed much of the self-help movement in general - seeks to have the subjective importance of diseases recognised by the doctor. This is stressed both (a) in order to utilise the patient's expertise as the sufferer of the disease as a contribution to diagnosis and treatment and also (b) to bridge the gap between the variant perspectives of doctor and patient, and thereby reduce communication problems and tensions in the relationship.

LITERATURE

Although a comprehensive list of women's health literature would be impossible, since new publications are appearing so frequently, it must be mentioned that book shops have been swamped over the last decade with such literature. These manifest a new approach to the reader, treating her as an intelligent equal, in contrast to many earlier - and some contemporary - advice literature which tended to assume the writer knew best.

The most prominent publication in this field has probably been "Our bodies, Ourselves", which was originally written by the Boston's Women's Health Collective (26) and was then revised for British readers by Jill Rakusen and Angela Phillips. (27)

An early British book was Nancy MacKeith's "Women's Health Handbook" (28) which was based on the political assumption that:

> The changeover from being a sort of barber's surgeon technician type to the present day doctor who makes moral judgements is very recent and very threatening ... women's struggle to control their bodies and their fertility is a political struggle.

The handbook has chapters on specific health problems such as hysterectomy, cancer and cystitis.

Not only is it necessary to see the women's health movement in the wider context of self-help and the whole women's movement, it is useful to understand in great detail the role of women in providing health care. These aspects have been reviewed by Lesson and Gray. (29) They note the prominent roles that women have had in the moves towards democracy and they "believe that the time is ripe for imaginative developments in the provision of health care for women, and that women will respond to such developments".

CONCLUSION

With its strength of feeling against the medical profession, the movement runs the risk of 'throwing the baby out with the bath water' and missing out on the benefits of mainstream medical expertise. There is, however, an awareness of this risk and thought has been given to analysing just what it is they wish to reject.

> Our sheer physical dependence on medical technology makes the medical system all the more powerful as a source of sexist ideology. They have us, so to speak, by the ovaries. All too often women have humbly accepted the ideological judgements ('you are sick, silly, hysterical, inadequate' etc.) as the price of whatever technological freedom they could wrest from the system. Now that we have come to take these freedoms just a little bit for granted, we sometimes lean too far the other way - rejecting the technology itself because we cannot stomach the ideological wrapping ...
>   But in our concern to understand more about our own biology, for our own purposes, we must never lose sight of the fact that it is not our biology that oppresses us - but a social system based on sex and class domination.
>   This, to us, is the most profoundly liberating feminist insight - the understanding that our oppression is socially, and not biologically, ordained. To act on this understanding is to ask for more than 'control over our own bodies'. It is to ask for, and struggle for, control over the social options available to us, and control over all the institutions of society that now define these options.

This is summed up in the key statement "... self-help, which emphasises self-examination and self knowledge, is an attempt to seize the technology without buying the ideology". (30)
What has the movement achieved? It is, of course, very difficult to trace precise paths of cause and effect but there undoubtedly have been

changes in medical attitudes. These reflect the
changing climate of opinion, to which the women's
health movement has contributed. Hospital practices
have changed in response to consumer pressure and
eminent doctors have spoken out for more humane and
accessible services for women. (31,32)
   There are two, perhaps cautionary, remarks to be
made here. The first is that, although the feminist
view of medical care is gaining acceptance in certain
circles, it does not yet reach the majority of women.
It is undoubtedly only a minority of women who are
conscious of "their often untenable position as
recipients of male dominated medical care". (31)
   Indeed there is evidence that many of the
women's groups are transitory and there has been
little recent increase in overall membership or
number of groups. (34) Here the health movement faces
the same problems as the rest of the Women's
Movement: that it is, in essence, a proportionately
small number of well-educated, relatively privileged
women.
   The second point is that the growth of women's
liberation has been accompanied by development of new
patterns of disease among women. If liberation for
women is only going to mean, being like men, then
they will run the risk of suffering the same health
problems as men.
   It would seem, however, that the Women's
Movement has the ingredients for becoming an
effective force in some fields of health:
1.   It works on the principle of patients taking
responsibility for themselves and for the groups and
organizations in which it partakes.
2.   It seeks to disseminate information and lend
confidence, thereby encouraging frightened or
embarrassed women to go for treatment.
3.   It wants to make women aware of the way their
body works - and thereby lends importance to women
feeling physically well and fit, putting the accent
on health, rather than sickness.
   The movement's energy lies in the fusion of the
age-old, deeply felt and yet unvoiced resentments of
women, with the new feminist analysis of male
dominated medicine. This new analysis has given women
the opportunity to bring to a level of consciouness
things previously felt only in a cloud of self-doubt
and confusion. It has provided the tools, a
vocabulary and a structure, which are enabling women
to translate their unease into alternative models of
health care, clear strategies and positive action.

NOTES

1. *Lancet* 1980 1.1284.
2. Marieskind HI. and Ehrenreich B. "Towards Socialist Medicine: The Women's Health Movement". *Social Policy* September/October, 1975. Vol 6 No 2 pp.34-42.
3. Coote A. and Campbell B. *Sweet Freedom* Picador. London, 1982.
4. Frieden B. *The Feminine Mystique* Penguin, 1965.
5. Oakley A. *Subject Women* Martin Robertson. Oxford 1981. p.308.
6. Marieskind HI. and Ehrenreich B. Op.cit. p.38.
7. Hornstein F., Downer C. and Faber S. Gynaecological self-help. In *Self-Help and Health: A Report* New Human Sciences Institute. Queens College C.U.N.Y., New York, 1976. p.67.
8. *Guardian* 22.10.1979.
9. Phillips A. *Woman, Heal Thyself* Guardian, 12.7.1977.
10. *Observer* 9.8.1981.
11. *Observer* 6.9.1981.
12. "Monthly Extract: An Irregular Period-ical." Published by New Moon Publications Inc. Box 3488, Ridgeway Station, Stamford, Connecticut, 06905 by Lolly and Jeanne Hirsch; Millie Alleyn. (Only complete set in England available in library of "Sisterwrite" Bookshop, 190 Upper Street, London N.1.) I.iii.p.2., 1972.
13. Ehrenreich B. and English D. *Witches, Midwives and Nurses* London: Writers and Readers Publishing Co-operative, 1976.
14. Ehrenreich B. and English D. *Complaints and Disorders. The Sexual Politics of Sickness* London: Writers and Readers Publishing Co-operative, 1976.
15. *Observer* 10.10.1982.
16. Tangri SS. *Population Dynamics Quarterly* 11. No. 4. Washington D.C. Smithsonian Institution, Interdisciplinary Communcation Programme, 1974.
17. Ehrenreich B. and English D. *Complaints and Disorders* Opus.cit., 1976, p.9.
18. Levin LS., Katz AH. and Holst E. *Self Care: Lay Initiatives in Health* London: Croom Helm, 1977.
19. Chertok L. *Motherhood and Personality* Tavistock Publications, 1968, p.24.
20. Friedman L. *Virgin Wives* Tavistock Publications, 1962. p.22.
21. *American Journal of Obstetrics and*

Gynecology 78. 661-5. September 1959.

22. Tunnadine D. and Green R. Unwanted Pregnancy, Accident or Illness? Oxford University Press, 1978.

23. Oakley A. Baby Blues. New Society 5.4.1979.

24. Kilmartin A. Understanding Cystitis Pan Books, 1973.

25. Williamson JC. and Danaher K. Self-care in Health London: Croom Helm, 1978. p.151.

26. Boston's Women's Health Book Collective. Our Bodies, Ourselves: A Book By and For Women New York: Simon & Schuster, 1971.

27. Phillips A. and Rakusen J. Our Bodies, Ourselves London: Penguin Books, 1978.

28. MacKeith N. The New Women's Health Handbook London: Virago, 1978.

29. Leeson J. and Gray J. Women and Medicine London: Tavistock Publications, 1978. p.202.

30. Ehrenreich B. and English D. Complaints and Disorders Opus cit. 1976. pp. 87-88,93,88.

31. Birth Control Trust. Day Care, Abortion and the N.H.S. 1980.

32. Kitzinger S. and Davies J. Place of Birth London: Oxford University Press, 1978.

33. New Society. Publisher's Advertisement. 'Women and Medicine' 1978: 45 No 831 p.523.

34. Wilkins N. Unpublished research findings, 1980.

Chapter Nine

EDUCATION AND PARTICIPATION

Why do we include a chapter on education in a book concerning patient participation? Because each depends on the other for its own progress; education enters into every aspect of patient participation hitherto discussed and participation is an essential factor in health education: the relationship is symbiotic.

We cannot hope to present an exhaustive study on the state of health education in Britain today: it is in itself a field of expertise demanding far more attention than we can offer here. But what we do intend is to draw out some of the aspects of health education relevant to participation and to explain their importance to each other. Health education means different things to different people and indeed many different terms are in use: health promotion, health and prevention; education for lifestyles; anticipatory care and health maintenance.

Is health education 'altering people's attitudes', or should the aim be to encourage people to 'make decisions' for themselves or is there some relationship between the two that is yet to be investigated? This important question posed by Sutherland (1) is a matter of constant argument and debate for all concerned with health as well as those directly involved in health education. Later in the same book, Tuckett, (2) in a paper entitled - Choices for Health Education, succinctly summarizes the position:

> there are three analytically distinguishable but compatible sets of reasons for health educating a population: to produce changes in beliefs and behaviour in order to reduce mortality and morbidity; to influence norms and values governing the use of health services; to

137

'oduce a general understanding of certain more diffuse 'health' issues in order to obtain a population who have a general understanding of health issues and to avoid certain forms of 'undesirable' or not directly definable 'unhealthy behaviour'.

An examination of the history of health education (1,3) and a review of its present activities indicates the changing philosophies associated with health education and the resulting differences and confusions in practices. It is not surprising that both those who are convinced of the need for health education as well as the sceptics ask - what has been achieved in the past and what is likely to be achieved by present activities?

IS HEALTH EDUCATION EFFECTIVE?

Health education has been around for a long time and yet there appears to be abundant confusion as to what it is, how it works, where it happens, who is responsible for it, and whether it makes any difference ... Most of us have the general impression that whatever health education is it is most certainly 'dosy and don'tsy'. It always appears to advise or admonish; it speaks to good habits and dangerous practices; or it extolls the virtues of checks and check-ups. In some form or other these views constitute a popular collage of beliefs about health education. (4)

Does health education work? How much is going on today? Does it have any risks? Such questions are easy to ask but less easy to answer. Accounts of education programmes will, however, be reserved for the subsequent chapters, while this chapter will examine some of the theory behind the practice.

THE THINKING BEHIND HEALTH EDUCATION

Although there are innumerable projects in operation, aimed both at management and prevention of existing health problems for the general public and in spite of the fact that both in Britain and the United States of America there exists bodies specially concerned with health education, there is still anxiety that there has been generally a lack of

138

methodological rigour characterizing health education in the past. Richards comments that,

> efforts have varied in terms of sophistication,
> intensity, quantity, quality and effectiveness.
> A variety of tactics has been used to inform,
> educate, persuade and cajole individuals,
> groups and communities to adopt particular
> forms of health behaviour. Some of these have
> operated formally, others informally and still
> others formally and informally. Inputs have
> been varied, and whilst enthusiasm has usually
> and initially been high, much of what is
> referred to in everyday terms as health
> education has been pragmatic, owing more to
> rule-of-thumb methods than scientific and
> objectively-tested techniques and strategies.
> (5).

Richards goes on to note that, although there has been a wide range of educative approaches, from face-to-face intervention to the use of mass media, all with varying degrees of success and failure, the reasons for the effectiveness of particular techniques and projects have often not been satisfactorily explained.

Such lack of retrospective analysis and evaluation has led, he maintains, to a lack of continuity. Richards concludes that there is a need for, "... good hard data to tell us how well a programme is meeting the purpose for which it is established, and whether it should be continued, expanded, cut back, changed, reproduced or abandoned." (5)

So health education needs evaluating. But in the process of evaluation there is the need not only to assess the method and medium of education but also identify the target group - the public, or specific part of the public at which the programme is aimed. So before any method can be decided upon, there is the groundwork to be done.

Increasingly during the past 20 years the social and behavioural sciences have made a contribution to the understanding of the relationship between individual beliefs and behaviour and have recognized the importance of social, cultural, religious and other factors in determining attitudes to health and disease, behaviour associated with health and illness and the use or non-use of health services. From this is growing a sound body of knowledge which should lead to new initiatives in health education, particularly if a multidisciplinary approach to health education research is encouraged.

If the current problems are to be tackled, taking into account the changing situation, a different outlook on education is required: one which encourages people, from a basis of knowledge, to choose between different paths of action, to make decisions and to participate meaningfully in both their own health and in the provision of health and related services.

GROUNDWORK

This can simply be described as the process of understanding 'how people tick'; what motivates them, what is likely to change their mode of life.

Green (6,7) has formulated a health education model distinguishing three sets of factors influencing behaviour. This framework is called PRECEDE (which stands for 'predisposing, reinforcing, and enabling causes in educational diagnosis and evaluation') and it draws attention to the necessity of asking what behaviour precedes each health benefit and what causes precede each health behaviour that must be addressed in a health education plan.

> Enabling factors include the availability and accessibility of specific resources necessary to take the behaviour in question. Predisposing factors include those social and psychological forces that cause an individual or a group to want to take or not to take the action in question. These might include attitudes, values, beliefs, knowledge, social norms, cultural taboos, and a host of demographic factors including age, socio-economic status, and family size. Reinforcing factors include those influences over which a health professional or the staff of an agency have some control in determining whether a given action on the part of the patient or consumer population is rewarded or punished.

This model was successfully applied to family planning health education in the People's Republic of China. It had the whole-hearted commitment and support of the community and its organizations and involved not only the message and the media to communicate with the public, but also the social institutions, the values of society and community resources. Further it has been concluded that,

> China's experience suggests that there is an
> element of universality in the social and
> psychological forces which enhance or impede
> change and in the educational components which
> facilitate the planning and development of a
> programme to influence health behaviour,
> irrespective of the social context in which
> education takes place.

Dr Nancy Milo also offers a set of propositions
for proposed strategies to improve healthful
behaviour by placing personal choice-making in the
context of societal option-setting. (9) The health
status of populations is seen as a result of
customary personal choice-making. These choices in
turn are limited by both the perceived and actual
options available to individuals, depending on their
personal and their community's resources, from which
to make choices. Most people, most of the time will
make the easiest choices, i.e. will do the things,
develop the patterns or life-style, which seem to
cost them less and/or from which they will gain more
of what they value in tangible and/or intangible
terms. The range of options available to them, and
the ease with which they may choose certain ones over
others, is typically set by organizations, public and
private, formal and informal. The more powerful the
organization, i.e. the more effective it is in
carrying out its policies, the more it affects the
options available to other organizations and
populations, whether or not these effects are
immediately perceived by individuals in their day-
to-day choice-making. (Hence the powers of tobacco
and sweet manufacturers and proprietary drug
comanies, manifested through advertising). Implications to be drawn from this framework are that it is
necessary both to make the health-promoting choices
easier and/or more appealing and at the same time to
diminish health-damaging options by making them more
difficult to choose and/or less appealing. An effort
at conveying more knowledge about healthful diets is
hardly likely to result in changes of eating patterns
unless it is accompanied by a combination of
appealing, healthful, low-cost, readily-available
foods - changes which require efforts by the
individual <u>and</u> the community public and private
organizational structure.
    Such examination of what influences and
motivates the target group is embodied in

Berkanovic's Health Belief Model (10) which:

> postulates that in the presence of certain cues
> or stimuli to take health action, the likelihood
> of taking action is dependent on the
> individual's beliefs about the seriousness of
> the health condition to which the action is
> addressed, his susceptibility to it, the
> efficacy of the proposed action, and the
> difficulties he may encounter in attempting to
> carry out the action.

Further, it is stressed that these beliefs are
linked tightly to the social structural position of
the individuals. This involves not only their 'social
networks' but the environment within which they may
find it is too difficult to alter their behaviour
because of the limited range of behaviours they can
choose. And it is here concluded that:

> Indeed, it would seem inappropriate to attempt
> to alter the behaviour of individuals living in
> environments that are hostile to preventive
> health behaviours without first changing the
> environment itself.

It was salutory to be reminded by Dr Leo Baric
(11) at the 10th International Conference on Health
Education held in London in 1979, that perhaps we are
as far from an accepted evaluative approach as were
the early health educators who claimed that it was
better to do something rather than to do nothing
because there was not firm evidence. Today, the
state of the art is better, there are reviews and
research in health education, and monographs on
evaluation, effectiveness and efficiency (12-14) and
rightly debate continues and there is an emphasis on
more and better research. However, there are few
studies that evaluate the effect of approaches that
seek to promote participation.

A NEW APPROACH

The scope of the present initiatives in education for
participation is illustrated by the objectives of the
National Centre for Health Education in the United
States. (15)
1.   Teaching people to use the existing health care
system more intelligently and more effectively.
2.   Teaching people to engage in more medical self-

care.
3. Educating patients to comply with instructions from physicians, nurses and other medical care personnel.
4. Helping patients to better understand their illnesses and to learn to minimise their need for medical attention.
5. Helping people to change their personal habits in such a way that the likelihood of illness is decreased and longevity increased.
6. Helping lessen medical malpractice actions by education of people about the limitations of medicine and by education of physicians concerning the patients' need for understanding.
7. Researching the appropriate incorporation of health education in all matters of primary patient care - when, where, and how best done, and by whom.
8. Educating practitioners - especially physicians and nurses - to become more effective educators of patients.
9. Promoting the further development of strong health education programmes in school curricula.
10. Promoting, demonstrating, and evaluating health education in the work setting.
11. Evaluating current health education activities and health education materials and disseminating the results thereof.
12. Helping people to understand the ever increasing costs of medical care and the personal and societal consequences of these costs.
13. Assisting people to make informed decisions about environmental matters affecting their health - ranging from water supplies to disposal of radio-active wastes.
14. Assisting people to make judgements when confronted with conflicting medical and other scientific advice.

Although many may feel that this list has a professional bias, with an emphasis on compliance and understanding of the medical profession's position, rather than a change of power associated with an increased participatory approach, it indicates the diversity of target groups - school children, the public, patients and health professionals, the diversity of topics and that clearly there can be no single approach and no simple method.

Many senior people associated with the field of medicine and health care in the United States have emphasized the need for an educational approach. (16-18) Massey, Dean of the School of Medicine in Connecticut has deemed public education to be the

most important challenge for the last quarter of the
twentieth century. Kerr White, speaking at a
Congressional Health Sub-Committee has listed public
education as the first essential element for a
national health policy. McNerwey, President of the
Blue Cross Association has called health education
for the public: "the missing link in health
services."

These all embracing statements are likely to
appeal to a wide audience but they must be related to
what has been achieved and what can reasonably be
expected in the next twenty years.

Massey (16) recognizes the limitations of the
past.

> It is not easy for us as professionals to take
> the matter of public education seriously ...
> the public seems to have gotten little useful
> information about health and doctors and seems
> to have gotten that badly ... Public education
> has not really been tried.
>
> Education of the public in matters of
> health needs nevertheless to be accomplished.
> Charging government with the task may be the
> best way of guaranteeing failure. Effective
> education should improve the health of the
> nation in a way and to a degree that nothing
> else could do. It should reduce the demand upon
> health services and reduce its cost of medical
> care and help to assure the necessary services
> are more generally available. It should make
> possible to provide for excellent services in
> response to an orderly and restrained demand.

The following goals might be considered:
1.   Everyone with reasonable understanding should
understand what is presently known about the prevention of illness. It is not much and it is not
complicated.
2.   Everyone should know that most illnesses, both
emotional and physical, are trivial and self-
limited, and do not benefit from medical care. There
are cheap and safe measures which people can use to
care for themselves during these short-lived
illnesses.
3.   The important techniques of emergency medical
treatment can be learned by almost everyone.
4.   The workings of the health system are complex,
but can be mastered.
Some would argue that the claims for improvement
in health and reduction in costs are optimistic.

While there is still uncertainty about the ability to undertake broad based and comprehensive educational programmes or the most appropriate methods to be adopted, the outcomes of such programmes may include a demand for a change in relationship between doctors and patients.

But education and enlightenment are mercurial commodities. Truly educated and enlightened people may not be satisfied with the acquisition of information and skills to suit someone else's purpose; they may desire to learn more, they may arrive at their own assessments and evaluation of a given matter. And as they become knowledgeable they may challenge, modify or reject the teacher's primary premise. Furthermore, it is impossible to engage in meaningful education without recognizing the impingement upon, and relationship to, fundamental philosophical, moral and value judgements. (16)

While at first sight this may be seen as a threat to the medical and other professions, and that conflict must be the inevitable result of these educational processes, there is evidence from studies on doctor patient communication, that education of patients may lead to an enhanced relationship and to better compliance (although this tends to imply obeying doctors orders rather than a partnership). Patients usually say that they appreciate the better understanding, are thankful to the professionals and indeed the professionals usually also are appreciative of the improved communication that has taken place. Professionals may have to accept that decisions by individuals (whether they are patients or not) and groups (with a specific health concern) may not be in accord with their medical advice, but that other factors, such as personal preference, cultural and religious influences, financial pressures or ambition may result in a compromise or a complete rejection of the professional advice. Another example is the choice of alternative therapies associated with decisions about side effects, pain, disfigurement, survival rates and risks. In the past the doctors usually exercised this decision-making, sometimes without the patient being aware of such alternatives, while now the decision may be made by patients and their relatives.

As is evident from studies on prescribing there

is considerable non-compliance – much of it not being known to the prescribing doctor. It would surely be better if patients are unwilling to take certain medications or have problems about side effects – to be able to discuss this openly and intelligently and that decisions by patients to discontinue medication are known to the doctors involved.

> A public educated to treat its minor illnesses and to recognize its symptoms will be better informed and so more inclined to question the treatment given by doctors. We should, I think, accept that if our patients become enthusiastic for self-treatment, the nature of medical work may change but the skill required of doctors will be higher. Ten years from now we will be seeing fewer patients but spending our time discussing with them diagnostic presentation and treatment
> options. (19)

The doctors and health professionals of the future will require great flexibility and knowledge of communication skills and educational methods – to be able to cope with those who wish much more active participation as well as those who wish to retain the traditional doctor patient relationship.

While recognizing the difficulties in health education, Massey (16) is convinced that not only is an educational approach worth trying, but that if certain changes to existing educational approaches were made, there is the possibility of being able to achieve definite results. Speaking to doctors he said that:

> Medical care or rather medical attention has been oversold, and the people have bought and expected the impossible. If we did it, then we can undo it, and it may be our moral responsibility as quickly as possible to get about the business of telling honestly what medicine can do and what it cannot do. Our patients have a right to know.
> Health education can be carried out through our existing institutions. It can and should be a part of the regular curriculum in the schools. Getting it there in proper form and decent balance is our responsibility. There is no reason why school biology should not be human biology.
> In the university, if science is to be

required for a bachelor's degree, it should be
the science of human biology. Just as no-one
should leave high school or college without the
ability to speak and write the mother tongue, so
no-one should leave without a reasonable
knowledge of human physiology and patho-
physiology.

Hospitals and employers - the latter as
part of their health plans - should provide for
continuing education in matters of human health
and in the ever popular science of human
biology.

As physicians we must first be certain that
what is presented in the schools and colleges,
and in our offices in no way violates the truth
and is useful information. Following our first
clinical dictum, it must do no harm. It should
emphasize health and not disease, and health as
a means for living and not as an end to be
sought for itself.

Second, we should reinforce in our
patients whatever true and important concepts
they may already have learned about health and
disease and we should seek out what they do not
know and help them to learn. For most of the
patients we shall see and during most of the
hours we shall spend in caring for them, our
most important task may be education. Whatever
a patient learns about himself from his
encounter with us, this may be the most
important benefit derived from his unfortunate
experience with illness.

These remarks addressed to American doctors can
be applied with slight modification to differing
health professionals in various countries. Such an
approach could be seen to set the scene for a new
participation in health, it could integrate much of
what is presently conflicting and would surely bring
rewards to both patients and professionals, but is it
an attainable ideal?

Although the distinction between individual and
collective responsibility has already been raised,
the World Health Organization (20) has drawn
attention to this in a slightly different way. A
working group on Principles and Methods of Health
Education has noted that health education should
activate the population to protect its health as well
as enhancing personal responsibility for health. The
community as a whole must take responsibility for
health education and must relate this to the other

147

main tasks for society. Individual and community participation in and responsibility for health are not alternatives, they must go together. However, specialists working from a scientific basis and with some form of organizations will be required to assist in such developments.

The next two chapters will examine some of the detailed educational approaches which have been linked to participation.

Categorization of these educational approaches could be defined by:
- the source of the material;
- the target population;
- the method of dissemination; or
- the nature of the message.

For simplicity the following chapters will adopt these categories:
(a) Information disseminated to the public in general – to provide information or advice about prevention, illness, promoting health or the use of services.
(b) Information given to people or groups with particular problems – often described as patient education. As in (a) this can either be about preventing complications of the particular illness, promoting health, or on the best and most appropriate use of services for the particular condition.

These two categories are not exhaustive (nor are any other more sophisticated groupings), but they allow the material to be conveniently brought together. There may be both official and alternative forms of education and an important component in either category may be the education of the professional.

It may be appropriate to end this chapter on general education with Massey's exhortation:(16)

> The commonest term we use in our language for physician, and the term by which we address him, means teacher. All of us who have to do with the caring for others are first of all teachers. This is our vocation for the last quarter of this century, to maintain health through better understanding and to prevent disease through knowledge shared with our patients. This is the high technology for the end of this century.

NOTES

1. Sutherland I. History and Background,

Chapter 1 in Sutherland I. (Ed.) <u>Health Education, Perspectives and Choices</u> London: Allen & Unwin, 1979.

2.   Tuckett D. Choices for Health Education: A Sociological View. In Sutherland I. opus cit., 1979.

3.   Baelz PR. Philosphy for Health Education. In Sutherland I. opus cit., 1979.

4.   Levin LS. Health Education: Moving to Center Stage. <u>Connecticut Medicine</u> 1975; 39: 631-634.

5.   Richards ND. <u>Methods and Effectiveness of Health Education: The Past, Present and Future of Social Scientific Involvement</u> Position paper prepared for the 4th International Conference on Social Science and Medicine, Elsinore, Denmark, 1974.

6.   Green LW. Towards Cost-benefit Evaluations of Health Education: Some Concepts, Methods and Examples. <u>Health Education Monographs</u> 1975; 2(Supplement 1): 34-61.

7.   Green LW., Kreuter MW., Deeds SG. and Partridge KB. <u>Health Education Planning. A Diagnostic Approach</u> Palo Alto, U.S.A.: Mayfield Publishing Co., 1980.

8.   Wang Virginia L. Application of Social Science Theories to Family Planning Health Education in the People's Republic of China. <u>American Journal of Public Health</u> 1976; 66: 440-445.

9.   Milio Nancy. A Framework for Prevention: Changing Health-Damaging to Health-Generating Life Patterns. <u>American Journal of Public Health</u> 1976; 66: 435-439.

10.   Berkanovic E. Behavioural Science and Prevention <u>Preventive Medicine</u> 1976; 5: 92-105.

11.   Baric L. Paper presented at 10th International Conference on Health Education. <u>Health Education in Action: Achievements and Priorities</u> London: H.E.C. and S.H.E.G., 1980.

12.   Tones BK. <u>Effectiveness and Efficiency in Health Education</u> Edinburgh: Scottish Health Education Unit, 1978.

13.   Bell Judith and Billington DR. <u>Annotated Bibliography of Health Education Research</u> Completed in Britain from 1948-1978. Edinburgh: Scottish Health Education Unit, 1979.

14.   Gatherer A. <u>Is Health Education Effective?</u> London: Health Education Council, 1979.

15.   Johnson RL. The National Center for Health Education in the U.S. <u>International Journal for Health Education</u> 1976; 19: 170-177.

16.   Massey RU. Educating For Change: The Next 25 years. <u>Connecticut Medicine</u> 1976;

40: 713-717.

17. White K. Quoted by Massey, opus cit., 1976.

18. McNerwey WJ. Quoted by Massey, opus cit., 1976.

19. Smith T. Book review. British Medical Journal 1979; 2: 199.

20. World Health Organization. Principles and Methods of Health Education Report of a Working Group. EURO REPORTS, Series 11. Copenhagen: W.H.O., 1979.

Chapter Ten

EDUCATION FOR HEALTH

Providing general information to the public has been
the traditional role of health education but there is
evidence of new methods and approaches being
introduced. While there is still use of approaches
based on the preventive medical model, associated
with exhortations to individuals to stop or reduce
harmful activities and to adopt health promoting
activities, more recently the emphasis has moved to
an educational approach which encourages individuals
to make meaningful choices and decisions related to
health. This will also involve decisions on the use
of services and participation in decisions
previously regarded as within the professional
domain.
    The examples in this chapter will illustrate
both the individual and collective approach to health
education although the majority appear to be
primarily aimed at encouraging change in individual
behaviour. Some can also be used by groups or
collectives seeking to promote social change.
    The routine health education programmes used in
schools and the mass media health education
approaches will receive brief mention only, as they
are not particular examples of participation.
Reference will be made when they are changing towards
a more participatory approach. It is salutory to be
reminded of the very limited success that has been
achieved even in the areas that have received most
attention. Referring to the World Health
Organization's "Smoking Control Day" on 7th April
1980, a leader in the British Medical Journal, (1)
entitled "The Avoidable Holocaust - Past
Irresponsibility", points to the failures, including
lack of government support - "We have now had
undoubted objective facts about cigarette smoking
and disease for twenty years, and yet our rulers,

charged with responsibility for public health, have done virtually nothing."

THE MEDIA IN GENERAL

The daily and weekly press, magazines, radio and television have over the years produced many features on all aspects of health, disease, care and cure - most designed to be of wide interest. Some examine topical and controversial issues such as alternative medicine, drug addiction, alcohol, out of date hospitals, incompetent doctors and transplant surgery. Other articles and programmes are designed to provide information - often for a more limited audience - those having a baby, handicapped people or those who help the disabled.

A series such as "The Body in Question" run by the B.B.C. in 1978-79, proved immensely popular - a well produced informative documentary. While many programmes have aroused controversy and criticism from the medical profession, few have produced such united condemnation as the Panorama programme "Transplants: Are the Donors Really Dead?" (13th October 1980, BBC2). In the Medicine and Media page in the British Medical Journal the following week, the writer, while considering the 'Desacralisation of Medicine', an entirely progressive endeavour, and the attempt to remedy the present state of affairs by creating a sensible and well-informed public opinion as admirable, felt that this programme fell so far short that its net effect would almost certainly be to hinder rational discussion on this theme for a long time to come. Even worse, it was maintained, it was also a deception, in that it had pretensions to be taken seriously.

The leader in the same British Medical Journal (3) entitled "An Appalling Panorama" described it as a disgrace - a programme designed to cause the maximum disquiet.

> In a single night, Panorama has wholly destroyed all the efforts of the past two years to re-establish trust between television and the medical profession. But it is not only medical amour propre that will suffer. By the end of this year the transplant surgeons will be able to count the patients denied treatment for endstage renal failure. Already one unit has found - for the first time for many months -that relatives are refusing to consent to organs

being removed. When, as is inevitable, patients die, the B.B.C. will have those deaths on its conscience.

If relatives do refuse, and if the public do tear up their donor cards, the ability of the media to influence, and the effect of one single programme will be shown. Will it nullify much of the steadily built up effort to encourage people to sign donor cards? How will it relate to the almost simultaneously published lengthy and dramatic account of heart transplantation in the Sunday Times? (4) The immediate pressure produced an additional Panorama which aimed to present a more balanced statement - but what of the long term?

THE OPEN UNIVERSITY AND
SPECIFIC EDUCATIONAL PROGRAMMES

A more directly educational role is undertaken by the Open University in conjunction with the media. In addition to courses on topics such as disability and social services, which form academic modules, the Open University has designed courses aimed at a more general audience. "The Pre-School Child", "The First Year of Life" and "Health Choices" have been prepared in conjunction with the Health Education Council and a number of advisers as part of a continuing education programme and not as part of the normal undergraduate courses. The use of an integrated approach involving a number of organizations and the media skills developed by the Open University is likely to provide the basis for further exciting and useful developments. The Good Health Guide (5) which forms a major part of the "Health Choices" course is also available on its own through bookshops.

A very different approach has been that of allowing organizations the professional facilities of the media, without the usual professional editing and censorship, to describe their work. Open Door and Grapevine: The Self-Help Show are examples of this innovative approach. Self-help organizations are encouraged to put out their own material, their propaganda and appeals to a larger audience on national television - usually at a non-peak viewing period, but still an opportunity not previously available. Anyone interested in details about something presented in 'Grapevine' could write to the B.B.C. for addresses and additional information sheets which explained in greater depth, the ideas already presented.

153

LOCAL RADIO

This seems to provide a special opportunity for designing programmes in local health topics and health services. One example (6) indicates the possibilities which could be more generally explored. Following a radio phone-in programme and a number of interviews in town streets to determine the topics of greatest concern to the local population, a series of eight, twenty-minute programmes on health education were devised. Preliminary evaluation of these programmes indicated that they were successful in imparting knowledge and that the information was welcome.

An alternative use of local radio (7) was to encourage people to carry kidney donor cards by portraying illustrative accounts of life after a transplant compared with life on dialysis. In at least one area, a consultant surgeon in charge of an Accident and Emergency Department specifically approached local radio and recorded a five minute programme in an attempt to counteract what he believed to be the misrepresentation of facts on donor deaths which had been portrayed in the Panorama programme.

It could be said that the media have a prime concern for news and controversy. The risks of contraception, the pill or the loop, the side effects of drugs such as Debendox, the possible harmful effects of industrial substances on pregnant women, or the carcinogenic effects of asbestos, have all made the headlines or the news programmes. Do such programmes have a real value in alerting people who might be affected and in prompting the authorities into action or do they aim merely to fulfill an appetite for scandal, thus enabling viewers to feel satisfied that they are not the perpetrators of such errors and negligence?

The opportunites in the new Channel Four are indicated in the requirement for the Independent Broadcasting Authority to "ensure that a suitable proportion of the programmes are of an educational nature" and also "to encourage innovation and experiment in the form and content of programmes". Will there be the necessary pressure to see that education for health is included and will it be possible to devise new and effective material?

YOUNG PEOPLE

In Britain, as in other countries, efforts and resources have been deployed to develop and initiate new approaches to health education for the young – generally recognized as the key target group. As Reid (8) points out the change in the last twenty years has been dramatic.

> What is health education? How to keep clean and fit perhaps with an embarrassed look at the sexual behaviour of the rabbit, or, as it once was in teacher training, how to recognize measles and what to do when the drains were blocked?
> How is it done? Traditionally, a few homilies in Assembly, visits from the temperance society and the Drugs Squad and perhaps a C.S.E. for the less able?
> No one will recognize it now – health education is suddenly the focus for reports, working parties, curriculum projects and resources with at least £3m spent annually on its support by health and education authorities.

The Schools Council and the Health Education Council have both been responsible for developing new curricula, educational approaches and materials for different age groups. Specialist organizations such as the Teachers Advisory Council on Alcohol and Drug Education have also contributed to this new interest. In a working paper on the Curriculum 11-16, (9) it is pointed out that:

> All societies provide health education for their members. Attitudes to health are part of the value system of any society. They are developed in numerous subtle ways by the family, by peer groups, by clubs, societies and religious organizations, by the schools, by the publicity media, by the provision and siting of health and social services, by laws and their enforcement and by the behaviour of people who are emulated.
> These attitudes need to be considered, discussed and evaluated within the school curriculum. Health is not a Utopian concept, but an important part of the ability to function and to adapt positively within the real world. The knowledge, skills and attitudes which

contribute to it are necessary for everyone and need to be acquired before leaving school.

Health education is part of <u>the education of the individual</u>. It is relevant to a consideration of <u>education for family life and living in society</u> ... It is part of education <u>for the world of work</u> ...

Health education is a continuing need for everyone, but it must respond to changing and varying needs. It will therefore vary from time to time and from place to place. Each school will meet the perceived needs of its pupils in its own way; it is important that this response should be planned and co-ordinated, providing all pupils with an integrated and continuous programme carefully related to each stage of the personal development of both boys and girls.

Research has played an important part. Balding (10,11) has shown the gap between what pupils and teachers consider to be interesting, important and relevant, and approaches such as this combined with educational skills will clarify for a teacher the aims and objectives of an educational programme and will allow for greater pupil participation and produce relevant and acceptable learning.

CONTINUING GENERAL HEALTH EDUCATION

In most countries the mass media have been the focus for "official" health education. One or more government organizations, or nationally sponsored voluntary organizations have provided authoritative, yet usually non-controversial health education by means of special campaigns. These may involve television, radio, posters, leaflets and the press and are aimed at wide audiences. These national activities may be supplemented or applied to particular local needs by local organizations or institutions. There may be simulataneous actions which reinforce the campaign, such as the introduction of non-smoking in cinemas and trains.

However, these campaigns are beginning to change as is seen by the Look After Yourself Campaign from the Health Education Council. It seeks to encourage participation in health promoting activities, emphasising fitness, the importance of exercise and appropriate diet. While discouraging unhealthy habits such as smoking, this is seen as part of the overall positive message. It shows how simple changes can lead to an improved quality of life and that being fitter can be fun - indeed humour was an important feature of the campaign. In 1978, in the first campaign (it has since been repeated) following press and T.V. coverage, including associated programmes, over a million people sent for a 'Health Pack'. In the monitoring of the campaign, there was evidence amongst other changes of an increase in regular exercise and the use of reducing diets. (12)

A similar campaign started in Scotland - "Fit for Life" is designed to run for twenty years. It is organized by the Scottish Health Education Group and the Scottish Sports Council, with the support of the Royal College of Physicians of Edinburgh. Walking, jogging, cycling and swimming are being particularly encouraged. Many local authorities and industrial organizations have started related 'Fit for Life' programmes and fitness 'casebooks' have been designed for use with the campaign. Thus there is a co-ordinated initiative at national and local level using mass media and individual packs. The title of one publication "Help Yourself to Health" (13) clearly indicates the message.

Adult education as organized by extra-mural departments of universities, colleges, local authorities, departments of adult and further education, Workers' Educational Association, and voluntary organizations has changed dramatically during the past ten years. Some areas have pioneered a 'community college' which brings together on the one site the learning facilities for all ages and needs of a community. While traditional courses on pottery, local archaeology and car maintenance still exist, many day-time and evening classes now include health and health related topics such as:

> Approaches to childbirth
> Whose business is health?
> Structure and politics of health provision
> Pre-retirement
> Food, diet and health
> The human body
> Alternative medicine
> The practical needs of children
> Mental illness
> Drugs and society
> Stress and the individual.

Both traditional didactic methods as well as more participatory approaches are used. With a greater emphasis on the local community, starting 'where people are at' it may be easier to make health a relevant and vital issue.

This will inevitably uncover root causes of bad health such as tedious and stressful jobs, unenviable working environments, poor housing and low income and unavoidably enter the political arena. But since the evidence (14-16) that such poor living conditions are causal factors in poor health and obvious inequalities in health, then, this would seem to be a reasonable and necessary step.

EDUCATION AIMED AT SELECTED GROUPS

Here the aim is to provide a particularly relevant message to a group with a specific need or problem. The message is usually disseminated widely but it is anticipated that it will be selectively accepted by the appropriate group. This message may sometimes be supplemented by those (professionals or non-professionals) working with the group, through discussion or additional material.

Long established examples are the various messages directed at pregnant women, with more recent examples being in the field of screening for cervical cancer and encouragement for women to attend for breast screening or to undertake regular self-examination of the breasts. Perhaps the best known example is the work of Dr Spock (17) first published in 1946 and still a major source of help and advice to parents of young children.

An unusual experiment using telephone dialling is the Can-Dial Scheme (18) with a collection of thirty-six tapes on health education and cancer control. In its first year of operation it had 30,000 enquiries. A similar approach providing anonymous information on the topic of venereal disease has been reported from Holland. (19)

DENTAL HEALTH EDUCATION

It has long been recognized that the vast majority of dental disease is potentially preventable and that the main responsibility for prevention lies with the individual and relates to dietary habits and oral hygiene. This must be regarded as one of the main challenges to health education and although much effort has been directed to education in childhood, the enormous amount of dental disease and suffering, particularly in the Western World, points to a failure to achieve change in individual behaviour.

In Cambridge, the Dental Health Study, which is funded by The Health Education Council commenced in 1975. (2) It has been examining motivation techniques for improving preventive self-care skills in dental health, taking account of the total environment of high risk individuals. Two dental health motivation packages have been produced: The Good Teeth Programme for pre-school children and Natural Nashers for adolescents.

The work is now at the stage where national implementation is being considered and if this happens it will be the first time that any national programmes of dental health education will have been systematically developed and researched. (21)

Booklets on self-examination and self-care in dental health have been produced by many dental departments including the use of aids such as disclosing tablets which provide clear evidence of the effectiveness of self-care, toothbrushing and plaque removal and this seems to encourage better care. (22) An extreme example where patients are encouraged to practice self-examination of head and neck to detect neoplastic disease seems to be concentrating on a relatively rare condition when so much needs to be done for the commoner diseases. (23) It is likely that someone committed to good dental care would notice and act on any abnormality without specific training in the signs and symptoms of neoplasia.

It has been suggested that general medical practitioners(24) who have more contact with young people should be encouraged to participate in dental health education.

VACCINATION AND IMMUNISATION

The control of infections and communicable diseases in some of the countries of the world is one of the great success stories in medicine. The excellent work by McKeown (25) describing the changing patterns of disease emphasises the contribution of socio-economic factors but notes that associated preventive health measures played some part. Not all of the success of immunisation and vaccination can be attributed to educational programmes - indeed it may be that many who received these procedures, or who agreed that they should be administered to their children were not fully aware of what was being done, but submitted to professionals whom they trusted. Much of the success may have been due to dedicated and convinced health workers in clinics and surgeries.

The significance of dissemination of information is illustrated by the recent reports of adverse effects associated with inoculations, particularly whooping cough immunisation. (26) The resulting drop in uptake of immunisation, not only of whooping cough, but other associated childhood immunisations is well documented and has led to alternative schemes which omit whooping cough vaccine if this is requested by parents.

EARLY DETECTION OF DISEASE

Educational approaches designed to encourage the early detection of disease must be based on the belief that "earlier means better". It is not possible here to enter into the debate and to consider every disease where there is a possibility of some form of screening. The general principles which must be applied to screening are found in many standard texts. (27) It is accepted that early recognition, resulting from specialised screening, must lead to an intervention which results either in increased quality or quantity of life, and does not merely "eat into the lead-in period" - to a prolongation of knowledge of the disease with no effective intervention.

There are some rather worrying aspects of overenthusiastic acceptance of screening - indeed instead of professionals seeking to educate a reluctant public, there is now evidence of the public seeking services from reluctant professionals. The demand for well-women screening is one example, (28) although there is still debate as to the effectiveness of screening procedures, the best methods, intervals between screening and priority age and social class groups - more especially with breast cancer than cervical cancer. (29-30) While considerable educational effort has therefore been devoted to encourage breast self-examination, less attention has paid to informing people about the nature of intervention if cancer is discovered. (31) Many women's groups are now seeking to redress this with a more comprehensive educational approach to the entire problem and not just one part of it.

The development of Do-It-Yourself Blood

Pressure Machines (32) has added a new dimension to early detection of abnormal physiology as well as providing a simple means for those with hypertensive disease of monitoring their progress and the effect of therapy. The machines are relatively inexpensive and can be bought for the home or can be used in some shops or department stores. There do not appear to be any difficulties in understanding the instructions or reading the results.

While it has long been accepted that individuals can and should monitor their weight - norms are readily available, considerable concern has been expressed about blood pressure monitoring - as leading to anxiety or being difficult to interpret what should be regarded as normal. Is this something which should be retained by the medical profession, who may be rather reluctant to carry out widespread screening or does this provide a useful means of bringing some people to professional care at an early stage and thus lead to a reduction in the complications of untreated hypertension? Although there is still some uncertainty (33) about when to intervene in mild hypertension, and the effectiveness of alternatives to drugs, such as relaxation or dietary restriction of salt, it has not yet been suggested that patients should initiate therapy.

From efforts like these, where there is informed public participation, similar educational programmes may result, which will hopefully lead to a reduction of the effects of additional serious illnesses.

DETAILED EDUCATIONAL PROGRAMMES

General health education programmes for children and adults in schools or in the mass media, have been careful to provide information that is recognized to be broad based and generally acceptable and have not sought to provide too much detailed knowledge. This prevents any charge of trying to make individuals their own doctor. However, recently, some courses and publications, directly aiming to provide more detailed training, have gone some way to take over functions usually deemed to be the perogative of doctors or other health professionals.

One of the best known is that of Dr. Keith Sehnert, (34) who as mentioned earlier, seeks to produce a "brand new breed, the Activated Patient" - who is informed and takes an active role in all aspects of personal health care. In another example, it is the family unit which is involved in the educational process to produce what Pratt (35) calls the Energised Family. These and other similar approaches are based on the detailed knowledge of health and services which have been worked out by health professionals and have incorporated material which although possibly available to the public previously (but not easily available) had not been so in a systematic and ordered manner. They appear to have been well received, but are probably mainly used by individuals who would have tried to get this knowledge by extensive efforts but now find it much easier. The greater diagnostic and therapeutic knowledge, plus the enhanced confidence in the patient-doctor relationship needs to be evaluated to determine the contribution to health.

A rather more limited approach is seen in the field of first aid. There has been a renewed interest in the teaching of first aid in Britain, possibly partly encouraged by government proposals on first aid training and the aim to extend the role of first aiders in industry. (36) An unusual study (37) has examined the attempt to provide comprehensive training in first aid to an entire community to see if this could result in a long term effect. At present preliminary results have shown a reduction in recorded accidents and it may be that a course like this not only produced detailed knowledge of emergency care, but an enhanced awareness of health and prevention.

An even more specific programme has been the attempt to disseminate information and skills in cardio-pulmonary resuscitation. (38) The aim is to reduce the number of deaths from heart attacks, drowning, suffocation or electrocution. Although some doubts have been expressed about this narrow objective - will the people trained be able to recognize the indications and appreciate the few risks? - this approach has been supported by the Working Party of the Royal Colleges of Physicians and the British Cardiac Society. (39) The specific skills can be learned but there are relatively few opportunities for people to practise them. There is a suggestion (40) that there is improved survival of patients with cardiac arrest when resuscitation is started by passers-by. It is not yet certain how useful such limited skills are or if it would be better to include them as part of an overall programme of education in health, self-care, emergency care and use of health services. Perhaps the ultimate in preparedness for treatment of possibly preventable deaths is the suggestion that every home of a person at risk (and the definition of who would be included would be difficult) should have a portable defribrillator next to the television set. (41)

DISSEMINATION OF A NEW TECHNIQUE

One of the major causes of death in children in the developing countries is from dehydration associated with diarrhoea, which in turn is related to a number of infections. In many countries, especially in the rural areas, there is no easy access to hospital for orthodox medical treatment using special hospital facilities. The recognition that there is a simple, safe, proven effective treatment which does not require hospital facilities is one of the major breakthroughs in treatment. (42)

"If diarrhoea is to be treated early, common barriers to treatment must be removed. This means that treatment must be easily available and inexpensive and it must be effective". There is as Pierce and Hirschorn point out an answer - "oral fluid - a simple weapon against dehydration" and as a result of the remarkable results noted in trials, the World Health Organization published a guide on the subject for the use of medical assistants and other primary health workers. The materials required and the appropriate instructions are now being given to mothers in rural areas, often by the traditional midwife as well as the other trained primary care workers. Thus a mother is ready to treat a child when the illness begins, without the need for immediate recourse to a health worker.

The dissemination and application of this simple technology may prove to be one of the most significant measures to reduce deaths in children on a worldwide basis.

THE DEFINED NEEDS OF A POPULATION

One aspect of distinct and possibly differing health needs is where there is an ethnic minority. A paper by Rowell and Rack (43) shows how in an English city, specific methods have been adopted to meet such needs, but the authors consider that their suggestions must be regarded as only a beginning.

The following health problems have been defined:
1.   Diseases which are present before arriving in

Britain.
2. Ill health following migration:
Physical adaptation and exposure to new infections
Diet and nutritional disorders
Injury risks
Emotional and Psychological Problems and 'Social Health'
3. Reliance on traditional systems of health care (this may present a genuine health problem or may be wrongly thus perceived, owing to the cultural bias of Western observers. As stated before, the keynotes must be sound evaluation and a recognition of the importance of starting 'where people are at'.)
4. Inability or unwillingness to make use of English Health Services.
From this definition of the situation, action to date has included:
(a) Medical screening of all immigrants on arrival.
(b) Employment of interpreters and special social work aides plus the production of leaflets for patients.
(c) Close liaison between the Area Medical Officer or his staff and members of the Asian Community. The establishment of a Health and Welfare Panel by Bradford Community Relations Council which has mounted special educational projects, e.g. rickets. The Transcultural Psychiatry Unit at a local hospital runs regular workshops for members of different disciplines.
(d) Seminars on Asian Culture for hospital staff and Urdu classes for professional workers.
(e) Co-ordinated efforts by the Education Department for both children and adults, including home tutors and neighbourhood language classes. Certain health education material has been included.
(f) Specialised case-workers employed by the Social Services Department.
(g) A co-ordinating and consulting function has been undertaken by the Area Health Education Unit which has produced a collection of teaching material in various Asian languages.
Despite these efforts they consider that further attention has to be directed towards the education of the health professional; an encouragement to the immigrant communities to make more effective use of health services and more education on self-care.
This seems to present a good model of how, by bringing people together, encouraging participation and clarifying needs, problems can be tackled.

Educational approaches are included and related to additional service provisions. The costs can be low as frequently the main task is to co-ordinate existing services, provide some additional training and to maximise existing effort. This is a framework which could be adapted to differing needs.

THE GENERAL PRACTITIONER

Reference has already been made on several occasions to the part in education which could be played by the General Practitioner and other members of the primary care team. The potential in each primary care consultation may be considered (44) to include four elements:

> Management of presenting problems;
> Modification of help-seeking behaviour;
> Management of continuing problems;
> Opportunistic health promotion.

While these are valuable opportunities for prevention, they are inevitably limited to those who consult. If there is to be an outward reaching approach orientated to the practice population; rather than to the individual, an efficient record system which enables staff to define age, sex and diagnostic groups is essential.

Tyser (45) in an excellent review notes the key role of the primary care team.

> The opportunity to work with a defined population presented in general practice, makes the primary care team an explicit instrument for the improvement of the nation's health by creating a better informed public on matters of healthy living.

This may be achieved if

> general practitioners make use of the profess-
> ional expertise and advice of the health
> education officer and, with their attached
> health visitors, undertake health education
> both in the one-to-one relationship and on a
> group basis.

The opportunities for health education are well documented but there is much less information as to what use is made of these opportunities, or an evaluation of these activities. As Pike (46) has said "It is during the consultation that family doctors have an almost unrivalled opportunity to communicate ideas about healthy living" - but do they? and how is it received? While much of the educational approach in general practice has been aimed at individuals or groups with a specific problem or need (or to parents of children with problems) and this will be considered under patient education, several attempts have been made to promote general health education - often with an emphasis on the use of services. Some studies have concentrated on groups, such as mothers of young children, while others have made educational materials generally available or invited members of the practice to attend lectures, discussions etc. The aim has usually been to encourage good self-care for self-limiting conditions. Experiments with telephone dialing in the surgery waiting room, for a series of recorded messages or rotating advertising machines have reported considerable patient interest. With the advertising machine, incorporating special artistically designed posters, patients could learn without being obtrusive (as was the case with the telephone) and it was felt that this appealed more to the naturally reticent nature of the British public. (47)

As mentioned earlier, some practice association- ions have arranged various educational sessions.

If the recent Annotated Bibliography of Health Education Research in Britain from 1940-1978 (48) is indicative of the state of the art, it appears that there have been no large scale evaluative studies of significant innovations in health education in the context of primary care. Accordingly it is difficult to come to any conclusions at present.

PUBLICATIONS - GENERAL

It is impossible to begin to describe the range of publications available, their titles or their topics, although some specific examples will be given.

Some are general based, medical encyclopaedias (following a long tradition), others deal with a specific topic or problem, while still others tackle issues from a specific religious, political or group bias. The range of specific books is so enormous that no categorization is realistic and the few selected examples quoted here serve to illustrate the breadth and diversity. Similarly the material available in daily, weekly or Sunday papers, women's magazines and many specialized magazines would provide a fruitful area of study in its own right.

Some material is 'officially' backed, e.g. the booklets supported by the British Medical Association through the Family Doctor series - Heart Attack: Prevention and Treatment. (49) Others would seek to undermine orthodox medicine and the formal services or offer alternatives to them.

The Consumers Association (50) have an established tradition of presenting information not immediately or easily available to consumers in a comprehensive and straightforward way. This includes a number of aspects of health and illness and the publications are designed for the lay person who needs clear concise information or advice - particularly when there are a number of alternatives. Titles include:

Pregnancy Month by Month
Eyesight
Caring for Teeth
Health for Old Age
Infertility
What to do when someone dies
Avoiding Back Trouble
Which? Way to slim

THE GENERAL TEXT OR ENCYCLOPAEDIA

These usually concentrate on self-diagnosis and self-care, but frequently incorporate information on anatomy, physiology and pathology. Some books have an alphabetical list of symptoms, while others are more like an abbreviated and simplified medical textbook. A more innovative approach based on the flow chart is found in Vickery and Fries. (51) This book which was originally produced in America but later edited in Britain, in addition to some general highly readable material which includes a chapter on lifestyle and the possibility of change, uses a flow chart to indicate what should be treated and how, and when professional help should be sought. Most of the texts include a section on drugs and self-medication and some also describe the uses, abuses, indications, contradictions and the complications of prescribed medication. Sehnert (34) provides a very detailed text with special emphasis on procedures designed to aid self-diagnosis.

This aim of providing information for

responsible decision-making seems to be the most popular approach at present - encouraging people to look after themselves and to practice simple self-help with an emphasis on positive health and quality of life, e.g. Look After Yourself published by The Health Education Council and the series of booklets developed from the BBC TV programmes on this topic.

The Sunday Times Book of Body Maintenance (52) is one of the 'quality' productions associated with the National Press while an American publication, Personal Health Appraisal by Sorrochim, (53) similarly encourages readers to become aware of their health status, assess their habits, behaviour and life style and change them if necessary.

A review of one of the general texts illustrates the size of the market.

> To read and digest everything written on good health today would mean, it has been calculated, two and a half hours solid reading every night, followed by severe brain fatigue during the day.

The review recommends "The Best of Good Health" edited by Phillips and Hatch, (54) as an answer to the problem:

> A guide to all you need to know about good health with detailed information including diets, special exercises for every need. The quickest way to find a new and exciting sport - even a remedy for dull and greasy hair. An excellent manual for all the family.

Similar comments can probably be applied to many publications and presumably their mere existence shows that publishers know that they are bought - although there is less information on the use to which they are put.

SERVICES, RIGHTS, ALTERNATIVES

These publications (55-56) in general provide a list of alternatives with a brief description of each. They may be either an entire book or constitute a section of wideranging text. While some are primarily reference books, many discuss the rights of patients and indicate the best ways to achieve these, how to overcome barriers to obtaining care and seek to guide patients as to how best to deal with difficult situations. The Encyclopaedia of Alternative

Medicine and Self-Help (57) is exactly what would be expected from the title.

The Health Rights Handbook (58) provides up to date information and recognizes that despite increasing self-care other forms of participation in health care are required if patients are to have their needs satisfied. The message of the book is that "your body belongs to you and only you should decide what you do with it". It is designed for those who wish to have more control over the care they receive by knowing more about their symptoms and health problems and from a basis of knowledge are able to determine their rights and if necessary ensure that they are obtained.

"From Self-Help to Health" by David and Yvonne Robinson (59) provides a directory of self-help organizations, a description of their work and examples of problems within the scope of activity. Age Concern (60) has published "Your Rights" which is specifically designed for the elderly. The Directory of Pressure Groups and Representative Associations (61) lists 600 organizations covering a wide range of social, political, economic and cultural activities.

LOCAL RIGHTS AND INFORMATION

Allied to the previous category of publications, but possibly of greater use is the handbook containing detailed and practical local information and resources. An excellent example is "Health in Hackney. The NHS and how to make it work for you". (62) This was compiled and published by the City and Hackney Community Health Council. It is a 112 page free booklet and this quotation from the introduction clearly indicates its aims and scope:

> This guide is to tell you about the health service in Hackney, and to encourage you to use it. You may be entitled to a lot more than you think.
> Lots of people don't use the services they are entitled to, although there is a great need for health care in Hackney ... Some of our health services are very good. Some are not. Perhaps the money isn't always spent on the right things for this neighbourhood. If there are gaps, let's say so and if enough people say so, something will be done. This guide has general sections on doctors, hospitals, dentists and so on. Other sections are

especially for people who need the health services more than most of us; mothers with small children for example, old people and the mentally ill. We have tried to describe how the rights should work. We often say 'Go to your family doctor' or 'Go to your Social Services Office' although in Hackney this doesn't always get you very far. So we have also tried to give the names of other people who know what's going on and will be able to help you. If you have problems please get in touch with the Community Health Council. If we can't help, we probably know someone who can.

Another example is "The practice brochure: a patient's guide to team care". (63) As the author points out:

When people 'sign on' with a building society, an insurance company, or even a bank, such institutions make considerable efforts to appraise their new members of their aims, their quality and the extent of the services offered. Information in the form of leaflets and brochures are commonplace. This has become more necessary as the scope and facilities of such institutions have increased to meet the complexities of modern living. By contrast, a new patient registering with a general practitioner is lucky to receive even a card with the telephone number and surgery times, and indeed many patients get nothing more than a curt nod from a busy receptionist.

The production of a 22 page booklet in non-technical language describing the medical team, the function of its staff, how they can be contacted, encouragement to seek advice of nurses and health visitors directly, is compiled with some reminders about preventive health measures. It was liked and thought to be helpful by patients and from a series of hypothetical questions posed in a questionnaire to patients, it appeared that it would increase use of the non-doctor members of the team.

DIRECT COMMERCIAL

A number of products are produced by commercial organizations. One example is "The Dental Education System" produced by MacMillan Film Productions. A complete kit - projector and a series of film strips/sound cartridges is available. It is suggested that these can be used in the waiting room, at the chairside, or in the office, depending on the programme and the audience. They can be linked with the educational work of the dental hygienist or can be used in the training of dental nurses or other staff, although most of the material is designed for patient education. The programmes concentrate on general dental health education, some being designed for children, others for adults. A few aim to explain special techniques or appliances. Staff must decide on the value and potential use of these ready made products compared with material from organizations such as the Health Education Council or the likely greater value of producing their own educational materials.

Some materials are not so directly commercial although there is a commercial interest or backing: many of the food and drug companies support or produce a range of materials - some aimed at the public, others at various professional groups. 'Eating for a Healthy Heart' published by the Flora Information Service (64) is one example. The Milk Marketing Board may encourage a link between dairy products and health while a broader scientific approach is seen in Food, Health and Farming: Report of Panels on the Implications for U.K. Agriculture. (65) Professionals must, however, be encouraged to bear in mind that the main aim of commercially produced literature or films is to sell the product. Patients must be made aware of the distinction between health education material and advertising.

DISCUSSION

The full implications of these initiatives in education and participation are still not clear. Concern has been expressed by doctors in the medical press about the effects of the media - concern about increasing anxiety in patients and relatives, misrepresentation of 'the facts' and the risk of unbalanced programmes or articles. However, the weight of opinion seems to point to the greater anxieties caused by lack of information.

In many areas there are differences of opinion about the provision of care or treatment, or there may simply be uncertainty or absence of information. Heart disease is a good example. While some profess-ionals feel that the patient should be given a

straightforward didactic book that coincides with
their own views and makes it simple and non-controversial, others feel that the patient should be
encouraged to recognize the genuine differences of
opinion (which are likely to be made public anyway)
and exercise his or her own judgement, based on a
selection of informed reading. It might for example
be useful to give the patient and his relatives both
The National Dairy Council's "Coronary Heart Disease
- The Modern Epidemic" (66) and The British Heart
Foundation's "Facts about Cholesterol" (67) and then
participate with the patient and relatives in a
meaningful, free and wide ranging discussion. Even if
professionals do not actively recommend particular
books, it is incumbent on them to be familiar with
the range of current and popular publications, so
that they can take part in discussion initiated by
patients.

Nutrition seems to be one area where there has
been a failure to produce either national policies
(68-69) with related educational programmes or
indeed any significant local initiatives. This is
despite considerable agreement on general principles
and a widespread public interest. The interest in
fibre by both professionals and the public is a
fascinating example of dietary change. (70)

There is a clear need to undertake evaluative
studies (71) of the sorts of programmes that have
been described and for a wide range of pilot or
experimental studies to be initiated.

Obviously the media can be involved in every
aspect of health, illness and care. They can
highlight tragedy or the dramatic solution to a
frightening disease; they can point to the failures
or successes of health care at either a national or
local level; or they can champion the cause of an
individual. This may take the form of a carefully
researched documentary, a thrilling play, a radio
phone-in or a sensational article in a newspaper.
Much depends on the interest, knowledge and attitudes
of those who plan, direct, research and present the
material. The end result may support medical
orthodoxy or it may blame it and advocate the value
of an alternative theory. It can encourage people in
their existing beliefs, deepen prejudices or it may
stimulate new attitudes and lead to altered
behaviour.

The media, however, are part of a wider educational process involving past experience - direct and
vicarious - the influence of peers and professionals
and the many other competing and conflicting

influences affecting both individuals and groups.

It is perhaps useful to conclude this chapter by returning to theoretical considerations after the many practical illustrations. Draper and his colleagues (72) in a recent challenging article have described three types of health education.

The first and most common is education about the body and how to look after it. The provision of information and advice on human biology and hygiene is vital for each new generation. The second is about health services - information about available services and the 'sensible' use of health care resources. But the third, about the wide environments within which health choices are made, is relatively neglected. It is concerned with education about national, regional and local policies which are too often devised and implemented without taking account of their consequences for health.

This third approach, he argues, is part of the currently moribund public health tradition and that limiting health education to the first two approaches may be "socially irresponsible". Only if health educators are prepared at local and national level to stimulate discussion, to show people how their choices are limited, to enter a dialogue with their community, to encourage members of the public to articulate their needs and to participate in policy making are they true to the tradition of their pioneering forbears and are therefore likely to be involved in a "social change movement".

NOTES

1. Editorial. The Avoidable Holocaust. Past Irresponsibility. British Medical Journal 1980; 281: 959-960.

2. Pallis C. Medicine and the Media. British Medical Journal 1980; 281: 1064.

3. Leading Article. An Appalling Panorama. British Medical Journal 1980; 281: 1028.

4. Sunday Times October 12, 1980.

5. The Open University in Association with the Health Education Council and the Scottish Health Education Unit. The Good Health Guide London: Harper and Row, 1980.

6. Turner RD., Brown JR. and England P. Medicine and the Media. British Medical Journal 1980; 281:40.

7. Medicine and the Media. British Medical Journal 1978; 11: 1291.

8. Reid D. Health Education - A Review of

Current Progress. The School Science Review 1978; March: 429-440.

9. Health Education Committee of H.M. Inspectorate. Curriculum 11-16. Health Education in the Secondary School Curriculum. London: Department of Education and Science, 1978.

10. Balding J. Health Topis and the Adolescent Nottingham: University of Nottingham, M.Med.Sci. Thesis 1978.

11. Balding J. Just One Minute - Health Topic Questionnaire London: Health Education Council, 1979.

12. Cust G. The Health Education Council and Its Work. Health Trends 1979; 11: 57-59.

13. Scottish Health Educaiton Unit. Help Yourself to Health Edinburgh: Scottish Health Education Unit, 1978.

14. Brotherston J. The Galton Lecture In Equalities and Inequalities in Health Carter CO. and Peel J. (Eds.) London: Academic Press, 1976.

15. Backett EM. Consumer Detriment in Health. In Why The Poor Pay More Ed. Williams F. London: National Consumer Council, 1977.

16. Report of a Research Working Group. Inequalities in Health (Black) London: D.H.S.S., 1980.

17. Spock B. Baby and Child Care New York: Pocket Books, 1946.

18. Wilkinson GS., Mirand EA. and Graham S. Can-dial. An Experiment in Health Education and Cancer Course. Public Health Reports 1976; 91: 218-222.

19. Schurman JH., de Haes WFM. Effects of the Automatic Telephone Answering Service on Venereal Disease in Rotterdam. The Health Education Journal 1980; 39: 47-51.

20. Dental Health Study. Whole, Healthy or Diseased Disabled Teeth University of Cambridge, Addenbrooke's Hospital Cambridge, 1980.

21. Craft M. and Croucher R. Preventive Dental Health in Adolescents Royal Society of Health Journal 1979; 99: 48-56.

22. Godin MC. The Effect of Visual Feedback and Self-Scaling in Plaque Control Behaviour. Journal of Periodontology 1976;o 47: 34-37.

23. Glass RT., Abka M. and Whetley J. Teaching Self-Examination of the Head and Neck: Another Aspect of Preventive Dentistry. Journal of the American Dental Association 1975; 90: 1265-1268.

24. Editorial. Doctors and Children's Teeth. British Medical Journal 1979; 1: 1231-1232.

25. McKeown T. The Role of Medicine Rock Carling Monograph. London Nuffied Provincial Hospitals Trust, 1976.

26. Department of Health and Social Security. Whooping Cough: Reports from the Committee on Safety of Medicines and the Joint Committee on Vaccination and Immunisation London: H.M.S.O., 1981.

27. Wilson JMG. and Jungner G. Principles and Practice of Screening for Disease Geneva: World Health Organization, 1968.

28. MacKeith N. The New Women's Health Handbook London: Virago, 1978.

29. Last PA. Breast and Gynaecological Screening. Practitioner 1981; 225: 633-640.

30. B.U.P.A. Breasts and the Importance of Breast Examination Facts About series. London: B.U.P.A. Health Promotion Centre, 1980.

31. Ulster Cancer Foundation. Reaching to Recovery after Breast Surgery Belfast: Ulster Cancer Foundation, 1979.

32. Lyall J. Be Patient with Do-it-yourself. General Practitioner 1981; 16 January: 44.

33. Office of Health Economics. Briefing No. 12 London: Office of Health Economics, 1980.

34. Sehnert KW. How to be your own Doctor - Sometimes New York: Grosset and Dunlap, 1975.

35. Pratt L. Family Structure and Effective Health Behaviour: The Energised Family Boston: Houghton-Hifflin, 1971.

36. Health and Safety Commission. First Aid at Work. Consultative Document London: Health and Safety Commission, 1979.

37. McKenna SP. and Hale AR. The Effect of Emergency First Aid Training on the Incidence of Accidents in Factories. Journal of Occupational Accidents 1981; 3: 101-114.

38. Lund I. and Skulberg. Cardiopulmonary Resuscitation by Lay People. Lancet 1976; ii: 702-704.

39. Joint Working Party of the Royal College of Physicians and the British Cardiac Society. Journal of the Royal College of Physicians 1975; 9: 2820346.

40. Eisenberg M., Bergner L. and Hallstrom A. Paramedic Programs and Out-of-hospital Cardiac Arrest: 1 Factors Associated with Successful Resuscitation. American Journal of Public Health 1979.

41. Friedberg CK. Symposium. Myocardial Infarcation 1972. Introduction. Circulation 45, 1972; 179-188.

42. Pierce NF. and Hirschorn N. Oral Fluid - A

Simple Weapon Against Dehydration in Diarrhoea. How it Works and How to Use it. W.H.O. Chronicle 1979; 31: 87-93.

43. Rowell VR. and Rack PH. Health Education Needs of a Minority Ethnic Group. The Journal of the Institute of Health Education 1979; 19: 3-19.

44. Stott NCH. and Davis RH. The Exceptional Potential in Each Primary Care Consultation. Journal of the Royal College of General Practitioners 1979; 29: 201-205.

45. Tyser PA. Health Education in General Medical Practice. The Health Education Journal 1975; 34: 3-11.

46. Pike LA. Health Education in General Practice. Community Health 1973; 4: 179-184.

47. Clarke WD., Davies M. Jolly BC. and Meyrick R. Health Education Journal 1977; 36: 100-103.

48. Bell J. and Billington DRD. Annotated Bibliography of Health Education Research in Britain for 1948-1978 Edinburgh: Scottish Health Education Unit, 1979.

49. Portal RW. Heart Attack: Prevention and Treatment London: British Medical Assocation, Family Doctor Bookelts, (one of a series), 1979.

50. Consumers' Association. The Which? Guide to Family Health London: Consumers' Association, 1980, (one of a series on health).

51. Vickery DM. and Fries JF. Take Care of Yourself. A Consumer's Guide to Medical Care Massachusetts: Addison Wesley, 1976.

52. Sunday Times. The Sunday Times Book of Body Maintenance London: Michael Joseph, 1978.

53. Sorochan W. Personal Health Appraisal New York: John Wiley, 1976.

54. Phillips P. and Hatch P. The Best of Good Health London: Pitman, 1978.

55. Inglis B. Natural Medicine London: Collins, 1979.

56. Eagle R. A Guide to Alternative Medicine London: B.B.C., 1980.

57. Hulke M. The Encyclopaedia of Alternative Medicine and Self-Help London: Rider Hutchison & Co., 1980.

58. Stimson G. and Stimson C. Health Rights Handbook Harmondsworth: Penguin, 1980.

59. Robinson D. and Robinson Y. From Self-help to Health London: Concord Books, 1979.

60. Age Concern. Your Rights London: Age Concern, 1979.

61. Shipley P. Directory of Pressure Groups and Representative Association 2nd edition. Epping:

Barker, 1982.
62. City and Hackney Community Health Council. Health in Hackney. The N.H.S. and How to Make it Work for You London: 1977.
63. Marsh GN. The Practice Brochure: A Patient's Guide to Team Care. British Medical Journal 1980; 281: 730-832.
64. Flora Information Service. Eating for a Healthy Heart London. (no date).
65. Report of Panels on the Implications for U.K. Agriculture Reading: Food, Health and Farming Centre for Agricultural Strategy, 1978, Paper 7.
66. National Dairy Council. Coronary Heart Disease. The Modern Epidemic London: National Dairy Council, 1978.
67. The British Heart Foundation. Facts about Cholesterol.
68. Oddy DJ. Perspectives and Strategies for Effective Nutrition Education. Proceedings of the Nutrition Society 1976; 35: 139-144.
69. Thomas JE. The Nutritional Component of Health Education. The Health Education Journal 1975; 34: 14-21.
70. Burkitt D. Don't Forget Fibre in Your Diet, To Help Avoid Many of our Common Diseases London: Martin Dunitz, 1979.
71. Sheiham A. Evaluating Health Education Programmes. The Health Education Journal 1978; 37: 127-131.
72. Draper P., Griffiths J., Dennis J. and Popay J. Three Types of Health Education. British Medical Journal 1980; 281: 493-495.

Chapter Eleven

PATIENT EDUCATION

Although the main emphasis in health education is generally considered to be to seek to prevent ill health and to encourage health promoting activites, another valuable, but neglected aspect may be covered by the heading 'patient education'. The aims are to enable those with particular health problems of both an acute and continuing nature, to make the most effective use of health services, to obtain maximum benefit from available treatment, to participate more fully in their own care and to learn to live with their condition so that they may attain maximum quality of life.

Inevitably a prime responsibility for this activity must rest with those who treat illness – doctors and nurses, yet there is still ambiguity over what could and should be done. In a book entitled 'The Rights of Hospital Patients' (1) Annas states the position clearly.

> The patient has the right to obtain from the physician complete current information concerning his diagnosis, treatment and prognosis in terms the patient can be reasonably expected to understand ... information for informed consent should include, but not necessarily be limited to, the specific procedures and/or treatment, the medically significant risks involved and the possible duration of incapacity.

The complaints by patients and their relatives about the lack of information, or their inability to understand what has been said indicates that effective communication is not achieved.

Is this because many doctors do not agree that giving such information is for their patients' benefit, or do they consider that this educational function is not their task, or has the information been given but it has not been recognized or understood by the patient, or do they simply not bother to give the information?

Doctor-patient communication is a subject which has been referred to on a number of occasions throughout this book. The failure by patients to understand terminology was noted by Boyle (2) and the many problems of communication between doctor and patient have been documented by Cartwright. (3) Her work showed that patients did desire to have information. More recently Dunn (4) in a study of patients after consultation with a general practitioner and Coutts (5) in her study of educational opportunities in the hospital ward setting, have clearly demonstrated (as have many others) the lack of knowledge about diagnosis, the causes of illness, prognosis, details and reasons for treatment and the wider aspects of living with a variety of health problems. Even very simple things like the nature and purpose of procedures such as an intravenous infusion were often not explained to patients. (6)

Despite the desire for information, many patients still do not ask the doctor at the time of interview (7) and this may encourage the doctor to believe that patients are satisfied and that his or her current practice is satisfactory. The recent comprehensive study by Cartwright and Anderson (8) examines the present position of general practice. Despite some improvements since the earlier study in 1964, the general message of the book is that there are still problems and that further improvements are desirable. Doctors were more likely than patients to feel that their patients were more knowledgeable and more liable to question whether the doctor was right. Patients appeared to have higher expectations and even among those who thought that their doctor was now better at explaining things, 14% were critical of the way he did so. Byrne and Long (9) from detailed analysis of consultations have described the 'styles' of general practitioners and this includes differing approaches to the transfer of information to patients. The wider aspects of doctor-patient (and patient-doctor) communication have been reviewed recently by Fletcher. (10)

Although, as will be shown in this chapter, there are a number of pressures which may be placed on professionals to become more effective in, and more concerned for, education of those with problems, it is likely that if there is to be an initiative leading to improved patient education, this must arise within the professions themselves or in the institutions responsible for their training. It is however perhaps salutory to be reminded of the legal position which seems to favour a conservative stance. Lord Justice Edmund Davis (11) outlined the common law precedents in Britain. He concluded that there is no strong precedent which places on the medical profession a responsibility to give information to the patient. In order to give a judgement against the doctor, the patient would have the difficult task of proving damages as a result of the doctor's withholding of information.

This chapter will not describe further the barriers to communication or the failures that patients perceive but it will look at some of the studies related to 'compliance' and the educational approaches that have been tried. It will also examine some of the educational approaches designed to aid self-care - both those originating from professional and non-professional sources. As in the previous chapter, it must be noted that the few examples cited can only give the briefest impression of an enormous and diverse field.

COMPLIANCE

One of the prime aims of professionals has been to reduce what they regard as the main problem connected with prescribed medication - non-compliance. (12) Non-compliance with medical advice is estimated to range from 30-50%. (13) This is drawn from many studies, mainly carried out by doctors and reported in the medical press. While initially it was believed that the traditional medical authoritarian model was all that was required, it is now well recognized that there is much greater need to examine the factors associated with non-compliance, such as the logical and illogical reasons that patients have for stopping or altering medication and the failures of communication on the part of the professionals. Eaton (14) and Haynes et al (15) have reviewed some of the recent research advances on the topic of compliance and examined both the theoretical and practicial aspects underlying this vast subject.

Stimson (16) notes that the problem is traditionally seen as "irrational behaviour" by the patient and that "blame" for defaulting lies totally with the patient. The recognition of the failure of this traditional approach has led, as Vaisrub (17) points out, to a concentration on the social context of the illness and on the patient, and that less indoctrination may lead to improved compliance.

Although it would seem to be desirable to seek to encourage improved communication which would in turn lead to improved compliance, it is necessary to be mindful of the following two questions: (18)

- Do we know that low compliance interferes with the clinical goals of treatment?
- Is it established that treatment will do more good than harm to those who do not comply?

A number of approaches have been designed to improve drug taking, to reduce error and to simplify what to the patient may be a confusing and complicated matter. In chronic illness which requires continuing and possibly life-long medication, which must be maintained at effective levels, the necessity for compliance is obvious. (19)

The desire and need for information on prescribed medication is well demonstrated in a letter to the British Medical Journal following a radio phone-in programme: (20)

> I was surprised at the number of people who were worried about the long-term effects of drugs and the possibility of their becoming 'addicted', particularly as the drugs most mentioned were minor tranquillisers and analgesics. More disturbing was the fact that many patients had no idea why they should still be having to get repeat prescriptions for these items after several months, if not years. The overwhelming flood of response I received was an indication not only of the interest the subject provoked but also of what appears to be a genuine gap in patient care somewhere along the line.
>
> Callers were generally shy to go back to their G.P. and not always able to get to the retail chemist. It does seem a shame that there is nobody to give a few minutes' advice or reassurance that could make all the difference between a successful recovery or a worrying course of treatment.

Some attempts at improvement have centered around measures designed to make medication simpler, more easily remembered and less confusing. In a study following hospital discharge Parkin et al (21) found that the two main factors leading to difficulty were the complexity of the prescribed drug regimen and the continuing availability of medicines prescribed before the current hospital admission. They were able to separate those who did not follow the drug treatment into two categories - non-comprehension and non-compliance.

Co-operation cards (22,23) which are kept by the patient and filled in by doctors at each consultation have been found useful in aiding communication in two ways - hospital and general practice, and doctor and patient, especially in conditions such as hypertension and steroid therapy where there may be frequent change in drug dosage. In steroid therapy there are implications for emergency care if the patient is suddenly taken ill as well as the importance of maintaining regular and even therapy. Repeat prescription cards are used by many general practitioners and the value of a two card system has been noted - one card for the patient to keep and one which is kept in the patient's file. Accurate information is thus available to both doctor and patient. (24)

The problems of the elderly who are on complex drug regimens are well known and numerous schemes have been tried to ensure improved drug taking - calendar packs, pill wheels and tablet identification cards. Some of these aids, e.g. pill wheels, appear to increase errors and studies have shown that personal discussion, follow-up visits at home and a self-medication training programme, supervised by a hospital staff pharmacist, while the patient is still in hospital, are of greatest value. All studies have clearly demonstrated the failure of simply discharging elderly patients with no preparation and no support. (25-27)

Perhaps one of the most important steps a general practitioner can take is to review regularly, repeat prescriptions in his elderly population in his practice. Tulloch (28) found in a practice, even with a lower than average prescribing ratio, that 10% of repeat prescriptions were unjustifiable and 19% equivocal. This step could be followed by one involving constant vigilance for adverse drug reactions. It is suggested by Martys (29) that during one year 40% of those prescribed drugs (or about 25% of the total practice population) may have had an adverse drug effect of some kind. This is higher than reported from some other studies, but includes less severe effects. If practitioners and patients are to cope with the complexity and risks of prescribed medication, effective education and communication seem essential.

The problem of providing simple accurate information on drugs was discussed at a meeting of the Medico-Pharmaceutical Forum in 1980. (30) A proposal was made at the meeting that some kind of national body should be established to produce these leaflets. There would be standardisation and general uniformity of the leaflets and efficient use of resources. Doctors, pharmacists, psychologists, consumers and others could all be represented on such a national body - which could start by designing leaflets for six common drugs and then do pilot studies to establish their use and effectiveness. But who will set up and who will pay? Some of this work is already being carried out by drug companies, but some participants at the meeting felt that such an important task should not be left solely to manufacturers.

The changing role of the pharmacist will be discussed in the next chapter, but examples of patient educational material either produced by pharmacists or by a team approach will be discussed here. Recently there has been a move to provide more detailed information to those who prescribe and secondly to the patients who consume the medication. (31,32) The aim is to accompany the prescribed medication with very detailed information - 'patient package inserts'. The main information includes: dosage, frequency of dose, duration of treatment, whether the drug should be taken before, during or after meals, whether alcohol, driving or operating heavy machinery should be avoided and whether there are any adverse effects requiring prompt action. As a leading article in the British Medical Journal (33) points out:

> in an age when unquestioning acceptance of professional advice is being eroded (and doctors who dispute or deprecate this tendency should recall their own attitudes to accountants, solicitors, and their children's teachers) younger patients in particular may wish to know how their drug works, how they will help their disease, why it is necessary to take them, and what adverse reactions might occur.

A clear implication behind any discussion of such written material is that it is additional to personal contact and does not replace discussion between patient and doctor or patient and pharmacist. The appointment of pharmacists with special responsibility for information and education is clearly a step in the right direction. One of them (34) has drawn up a list of existing booklets, cards, leaflets and information sheets produced by drug manufacturers. It is interesting to note that some of the leaflets are in different languages, recognizing the importance of ethnic minorities.

Patient education programmes (35) have been based on comprehensive written materials on prescribed drugs. The following advantages of clearly written specific information were noted:

- The patient can retain the instructions for referral at any time.
- Written instructions can serve as a common starting point for education by all health professionals and, by standardizing information, avoid conflicting directions.
- All patients receive complete, uniform information independent of the pharmacist's time and memory.
- The pharmacist saves time by reviewing only important points and answering questions rather than tediously repeating all instructions to each patient. Written instructions provide an efficient and economical method for the pharmacist to educate a large number of patients.
- Written instructions can reach patients whose prescriptions are mailed or delivered.
- Written instructions may serve as a basis for legal documentation that education was provided.

Table 11.1 lists the categories of information.

The Canadian Pharmaceutical Association (36) has produced for purchase by its members, Supplementary Information of Medication, for a variety of conditions. These have space for the pharmacist's name and make the written material more personal. It is noted that: "SIM's are not meant to replace pharmacist patient dialogue. They provide an extension to your professional service." Figures 11.1 and 11.2 illustrate these cards.

The key role of the pharmacist in education and the need for it is summarised in the conclusion of Fink's article: (37)

FDA conducted another survey to ask people: Do you read labels? Do you read labels on prescription drugs? Do you read labels on non-prescription drugs? It was concluded that only half of the people interviewed regularly read the labels of drugs which they use. Almost a quarter of the people surveyed did not know what the label meant, could not read the print because it was too small, relied only on the brand name, or simply did not care whether they read the label or not. Only one person out of six looked for information about side effects on drug labels. Only one out of 10 looked for precautions or contraindictions. Only 46% of the people regarded drug labeling as being understandable. Yet, the entire thrust of the Food and Drug Administration's regulatory scheme is to regulate the label so that the consumer will have enough information available to safely use drug products. In light of this survey information, the need for patient drug information is apparent. The pharmacist has a role to reinforce the drug information as well as to supplement it.

One final point involves the difference in the pharmacist role required between the patient who comes to the pharmacy with a prescription and the patient who comes to procure on OTC drug product. A prescription patient has already visited a physician and supposedly has already received an educated determination as to the nature of the ailment and a recommendation concerning therapy. But the OTC patient may not know what is wrong; the patient knows he has not had a bowel movement for 4 days, but not why. In this latter situation, the pharmacist's role is quite different from the role of the pharmacist with a prescription patient. With the OTC patient, the pharmacist has to actually assist the patient in determining what is wrong before being able to recommend a product. Helping the patient determine the nature of the disorder is important, if the pharmacist is to make a recommendation that will enhance the patient's health.

In certain areas where there is co-terminosity of pharmacist and general practitioner it has been possible to set up a two card system for patient and pharmacist with the specific intention of avoiding drug reactions and interactions. (38) Such programmes as have been described, must improve communication and awareness of professionals and patients, but do they improve compliance and do they lead to improved health? The answer to the first question may be yes, but the second question is still unanswered.

One of the key concepts in British medical practice is that of the 'personal doctor'. While many people have extolled the virtues of such a system, there have been few studies which have examined or explained it. In a study of compliance (39) in patients prescribed an antibiotic, it was found that compliance with the prescription was strongly associated with whether the patient thought that he knew the prescribing doctor well. As the authors point out, there are implications for improving consultation technique - particularly with new patients and for encouraging and enabling patients to see the same doctor.

SELF-MEDICATION

Considering the amount and significance of self-medication, which necessitated extensive description in chapter 5, it is surprising that there appears to be such a paucity of educational material associated with it.

Some information and direct educational material or advice is found in many of the publications described in the last chapter. Most of the general publications include information on treatment under the specific symptom or disease categories or have entire sections on self-medication. This is illustrated by the two well known books 'How To Be Your Own Doctor - Sometimes' (40) and 'Take Care of Yourself. A Consumer's Guide to Medical Care'. (41) Sehnert advises a much more comprehensive list of drugs than would normally be found in a British home medicine cabinet - as he includes a number of prescription drugs which would be used in appropriate circumstances by the 'Activated Patient'. In these books the use of both over-the-counter drugs and prescription drugs by the patient is discussed along with detailed information on the appropriate conditions, the proper use of drugs, side effects, storage of medicines, relationship to food and alcohol, and the indications for seeking professional help. This approach is quite different from the more traditional home doctor booklets or encyclopaedias which suggest care consisting of over-the-counter drugs and simple advice on sleep, nutrition and traditional home remedies. Specialist books may describe the indications and use of herbal remedies or homeopathic drugs.

The most extensive 'education' comes from the pharmaceutical companies that manufacture over-the-counter drugs. Television, radio, newspapers and magazines, provide the vehicles for extensive advertising and the advice that a particular product is the appropriate answer to certain symptoms or minor illness.

The relationship between advertising, communication and education was discussed thoroughly at the Workshop on Self Care held at the Royal College of Physicians in London in 1979. (42) In the paper introducing the topic, Cust and Wells (43) noted firstly that:

> if the lay public are to make informed choices about self-treatment, the degree of knowledge required may be grouped under four headings: medical diagnosis, conditions for self-treatment, use of home medicines and general health information.

Secondly, they emphasized:

> the use of a home medicine follows three stages: product awareness, product purchase and product use. At each of these stages there is a different information need.

For product awareness, most commonly the choice of home medicines is based upon family experience. For product purchase, while the majority of purchases are made by people who have used the product in the past, pharmacists are frequently consulted about the appropriate treatment of symptoms and the medicines available. For product use, the inner label (the outer container often having been discarded) provides the guidelines or dosage instructions, the cautionary statements and the advice necessary to ensure the safe and correct use of the medicine.

In a survey of the pattern of self-care in 1,000 patients, Eliott-Binns (44) found that sources of advice included relatives - (wives gave the best advice, mothers and mothers-in-law the worst), professionals such as nurses and chiropodists - (this overall group gave a surprising 6.7% harmful advice) and impersonal sources, such as magazines and local chemist shops (whose advice was largely sound). Home doctor books were kept long after they were out of date; one patient referred to a book written in 1894.

Table 11.2 shows the result of Cartwright and Dunnell's study. (45) These studies seem to indicate a limited role for advertising, but the importance of branding is well known and especially marked with analgesics. A study by Braithwaite and Cooper (46) has suggested that the effects are due to increased confidence in obtaining relief with a well known brand and that branding has an analgesic effect that interacts with the analgesic effects of placebos and active ingredients.

While the family experience is inevitably the result of many influences over a long period of time, it is evident that the responsibility of the manufacturers and the training and role of the pharmacist are key factors in improving education and information. Existing legislation already contributes to the printed information on the inner label. The Proprietary Association of Great Britain and individual pharmaceutical companies have been concerned to improve the information on the labels and this may include notices such as 'Keep Medicines Safely', 'Always Read the Label', to more detailed information such as 'For the Relief of the Symptoms of Flu' and notes indicating that if after regular medication for an appropriate number of days, there is no improvement, the medication should not be continued without the agreement of the patient's doctor. Such an approach could be linked either with local or national health education campaigns.

As was discussed in an earlier chapter, there is evidence that self-medication is widely and competently used by the public. It is unfortunate that there is little evidence from areas of the world, such as the Middle East, where a much wider range of powerful and specialised drugs are easily, if not cheaply, available, without prescription from pharmacies .

Self-medication in the United States appears to be generally similar to that in Britain, although the financial constraints of the health care system and the relative absence of general practice may encourage self-medication. There is strict control by the Food and Drug Administration of over-the-counter drugs and it is assumed that a drug can be sold over-the-counter if:

1. It is safe per se.
2. Adequate directions for use for the layman can be written.
3. Ancillary measures in conjunction with the drug are readily available to the layman.

4.   Indications for use are readily discernable to the layman.
It is required that non-prescription drugs must bear a '7-point label':
1.   Name of medication.
2.   Net weight, fluid measure or numerical count of the contents.
3.   Name and address of the manufacturer or distributor.
4.   Complete directions for use:
(a) the purpose or purposes for which the medicine is intended
(b) how much to take
(c) how often to take it
(d) when not to take it
5.   Names of the active ingredients in the medication.
6.   Warnings against misuse of the product.
7.   Caution concerning proper storage and advising when the medicine may deteriorate or lose its effectiveness. (37)

Paperbacks containing detailed information are available, but these are likely to be used for reference or by those involved in teaching or leading discussion. Examples are 'The Medicine You Take' (47) and 'Medicines - A Guide For Everybody'. (48)

In Britain, those involved in health education, at both national and local level, have been concerned to provide simple basic advice on self-medication. The Health Education Council in England, produced a booklet 'Treating Yourself' (49) in 1975 and the Scottish Health Education Unit published 'Help Yourself to Health' (50) in 1978. The latter, which included accident care and home treatment was supplied free to patients by their general practitioner.

These guides have been found to be generally useful (51) but as they have wider aims than merely providing information on self-medication, they might be of greatest use if they were part of a wider educational approach to participation in primary care, rather than isolated aids to self-medication. Although only a few examples have been reported, the possibility of the general practice or the health centre acting as a focus for such initiatives is being explored. Generally, the emphasis has been on helping mothers look after the self-limiting conditions that are common in young children. (52,53) One such study has been evaluated. (54,55) From practice records it was noted that for children under 16 years, over half of the new demands for care were concerned with six common symptoms - stuffy or runny nose, sore throat, cough, diarrhoea and minor trauma. An eleven page booklet was produced to inform patients about the meaning of these six symptoms, the appropriate type of medication and guidance on when a doctor should be consulted. The booklet did not appear to lead to increased knowledge, but 76% of mothers had consulted the booklet at some time in the year of the study and 28% had consulted it in the three months before the interview. The most important result was a fall in new requests for care for the symptoms described in the booklet. The authors concluded from the study that possibly what patients need to respond appropriately to common symptoms of illness, is a simple reference manual rather than an educational programme designed to increase their knowledge about the management of illness. However, it is necessary to beware of assuming that a reduction in professional consultations necessarily implies either improved self-care or greater patient satisfaction. As the authors note, there is a risk that such publications may be interpreted as discouragement to patients from 'bothering' their general practitioner with trivial complaints. More recently, the Health Education Council has produced a booklet on minor illnesses specifically designed for use by the general practitioner in the consultation.

In his analysis of lay-medicine, Eliott-Binns concludes that, although hitherto a neglected subject, self-medication: "may be an important part of family and community life." (44) Along with this recognition, Eliott-Binns wants:

> A plan for sensible and efficient training in home medical care, perhaps at school level, and further investigations into ways in which it might be extended to take away some of the burden of the National Health Service.

Commenting that only 25% of all illness episodes are taken to the doctor, the following questions were posed at a meeting of the Royal Society of Medicine: (56) "How good is this self-care? Is it not our responsibility as doctors to help our patients to make it as effective as possible?"

Pharmacists are also being seen as significant agents in the arena of self-medication. A survey of pharmacists found that over two days, twenty pharmacists in eight towns in England received 600 requests for medical advice. (57)

Webb (58) has emphasized the existing role of

the pharmacist as an adviser on non-prescribed medicine, while Harris (59) has studied extensively the role and functions of pharmacists. Both with prescribed and over-the-counter drugs there are enormous opportunities for pharmacists and all health professionals to work together to ensure the continuing safety and improved effectiveness of self-medication as a component of the wider aspects of participation in health.

PATIENT EDUCATION IN HOSPITAL

Education for improved medication is only one facet of a wider educational process designed to enable patients to live with their disease or disability and to aid them as they seek to improve their quality of life. Because it is considered to be less obviously 'medical', it appears to be a rather neglected aspect of care. Indeed, since it may not be felt to be any professional's specific responsibility, there may be an assumption that someone else will do it and in the end no-one does it. Frequently it is complicated by the failure of communication between hospital and community.

Coutts (5) in her study of gynaecological wards in Scotland noted the desire by patients for information on a wide range of matters, the opportunities missed by staff to give information, the low priority awarded to patient education and the uncertain responsibilities of staff for providing information. Information could be divided into three categories: nursing responsibility, medical responsibility and responsibility delegated from doctors to nurses. Nurses function well in relation to giving information to patients in areas they clearly identify as their responsibility, but this tends to be largely concerned with ward or nursing management. She pointed to the lack of doctor nurse communication and how this in turn may affect nurse patient communication and some ward sisters reported that they resorted to evasive action when pressed by patients for information. Uncertainty seems to lead to failure to provide adequate information to patients in hospital, about prognosis, future care, self-care and implications of the condition for many aspects of life.

The title of an article by Eardley and her colleagues (60) well illustrates the present state of the art: 'Health education by CHANCE: the unmet needs of patients in hospital and after'.

A later article involving Eardley (61)
indicated possible practical approaches to remedy
this situation. Patient education was to be based on
the wards, special programmes were to be devised,
tape slide material could be used and opportunities
were to be provided for group discussion. Similar
ideas were put forward by Richards and Kalmer (62) at
the first international conference on patient
education in hospitals, which was held in 1971. The
management aspects as well as the educational skills
were monitored and the importance of a team approach
involving staff with differing skills was stated. The
possible contributions that might come from outside
organizations and the role of the volunteer was also
raised.

A recent issue of 'Topics in Clinical Nursing',
(63) devoted entirely to Education for Self-Care,
indicates the increasing importance being attached
to this subject and the changing attitude of the
nursing profession to their role. In the editorial
they comment:

> From the unusually large number of articles
> submitted for this issue we must conclude that
> nursing is heading away from the strict medical
> disease model of patient submission to actively
> promoting the self-care movement by fostering
> direct initiative.

It is stated that the function of nursing is to
focus on the maintenance of self-care activities.
Individuals continually need to sustain life and
health, recover from disease and injury, and cope
with their effects. In the introductory article in
the issue, Hochbaum clarifies the distinction
between teaching people what the health professionals think they should know and devising
educational programmes that reflect what is
important and significant to patients.

> The patient educator must learn to suspend
> professional attitudes and habits, and enter
> into the patient's world, so that she or he
> comes to understand the patient's rationality,
> mentality and problems.

Throughout the issue in the papers describing
programmes for specific conditions, the key role of
the nurse is emphasized in patient education in
hospitals.

A comprehensive hospital-based educational

system aimed at patients, their families and friends, has been developed in the Soviet Union. (64) As regards patients, focus is placed on raising their level of knowledge about adequate health behaviour during hospitalization and after discharge, in order to prevent relapses, improve health and reduce complications. Topics covered include diet, physical exercise, developing resistance to the cold and giving up harmful habits. Individual and group activities are used at all stages of the patient's stay in hospital. The mass media supplements this approach through hospital radio and television programmes and the popular scientific literature from the hospital library. For patients' relatives and friends a programme of individual talks have been devised and special leaflets are distributed. Preliminary evaluation indicates that the system yields satisfactory results and is appreciated.

HOSPITAL TO COMMUNITY

The gap between hospital and community care is well recognized. It includes lack of communication between professionals in the two spheres, the lack of information to relatives and the often sudden and unexpected discharge of patients from hospital. These as well as the lack of service provision in the community are described by Gay and Pitkeathley. (65) The very serious lack of detailed practical information and help and advice throughout the recovery phase is reported in many studies on rehabilitation.

As noted in primary care, new staff attitudes are necessary for effective patient participation and the recognition that there is a special expertise in those who have suffered from a condition, that may usefully be handed on to new sufferers from patients with years of experience. New organizational structures are required if there is to be inclusion of patients and their relatives in the decision making process in rehabilitation - particularly involving alteration in the traditional hospital ward organization and staff roles. (66)

A number of hospitals produce printed material of various kinds to give to patients. Ellis (67) and his colleagues in a controlled trial of supplementary written information for patients, found that it led to improved understanding, recall and increased patient satisfaction and compliance. Such brief supplementary advice on illness and treatment provides the patient and his family with a basic document which could be used to encourage discussion and decrease family disagreement. It seemed to legitimate and facilitate discussions with general practitioners on issues which might otherwise have been considered to be inappropriate. They are of value to both patient and professional.

Some of the inadequacies of present booklets, given free to patients, have been noted in a study (68) of what is available in eleven different countries. While there were considerable overlaps in material, there were also important gaps. There was confusion, in heart disease, between prevention, secondary prevention and management, and the authors concluded that there should be one booklet covering the general principles of prevention and a series of booklets related to specific conditions and providing detailed management.

LIVING WITH CHRONIC DISEASE

In addition to providing detailed educational material for those with chronic conditions, in some conditions there is the possibility of patients being actively involved in the day to day control of their disease. In a symposium on self-monitoring, (69) three conditions were discussed - diabetes, hypertension and asthma, where there is the possibility of precise measurements - urinary or blood sugar in diabetes, blood pressure in hypertension and respiratory function in asthma. Improved techniques are enabling patients to undertake such review themselves, without regular referral to professionals and that these results can be used in the day-to-day monitoring of the drug regimen. Such participation appears to be generally welcomed by the patients and provides them with an effective basis for managing their own therapy and hence controlling their own condition.

Diabetes and hypertension are being used here to illustrate current practice. Since the introduction of insulin therapy, diabetics have been involved in the day-to-day monitoring of their therapeutic control through regular urine checks. The introduction of simple blood glucose monitoring apparatus (there are several different machines available) has provided an increased opportunity for patients to have regular and detailed information on their blood sugar and to alter their medication and possibly their diet and exercise accordingly.

Initial reports (70-72) suggest that there may be improved control, an increased patient satisfaction and the possibility of attainment of near normal blood sugar which may in turn lead to a reduction in complications. An additional value is that this technique may lead to improved control in early pregnancy, thus leading to a shorter time in hospital. (73)

Such technical aids to control, must not be considered in isolation and those responsible for diabetic care have established extensive educational programmes, including teaching aids, leaflets, information packs and have made use of the specialist nurse educators. Interdisciplinary teams have also been used to provide group and individual instruction and discussions for patients and their families. (74,75) A particularly useful source of information and support, particularly to the newly diagnosed diabetic, comes from the British Diabetic Association and patients are frequently put in touch with the organization during their initial hospital admission. The continuing importance of education - to reduce and encourage the early detection of complications has also been noted. (76) Effective education and participation can also be achieved in children. (77)

Hypertension provides another interesting example of education and participation in care. Unlike diabetes, where the effects of incorrect treatment are usually quickly obvious, there may be few or no initial symptoms and it is possible that the side effects of treatment may be more noticeable. A full explanation of the disease, its long term nature and possible serious complications may be necessary if there is to be continued medication. (78) The advent of simple and relatively cheap blood pressure monitoring kits has provided a similar opportunity for hypertension to that just described for diabetes. Initial trials suggest that patients find the process acceptable. (79)

Such developments in chronic disease care are exciting and show the importance of a good doctor-patient relationship and a partnership approach to care. Green and his colleagues (80) have shown the need for a comprehensive and intensive programme of education, rather than simply providing information. They noted the importance of providing training and education for the providers of care as well as the patients. Similar findings have been noted by Spiegel (81) in diabetic care. There is also a requirement for the general practitioner to have an efficient

record system to ensure effective follow-up of the
patients. (82) Simple leaflets produced by the
general practitioner (83) may aid communication with
patients and the value of shared records have also
been noted. (23)

In countries where there are industry or union
based health programmes, it is possible to use their
well developed communication and educational
approaches to encourage the detection and management
of conditions such as hypertension. (84) An unusual
experimental programme (85) based in industry, has
shown that employees with mild hypertension who, when
allocated to a biofeedback group and who received
training in relaxation and management of stress (both
experimental and control groups had received simple
health education literature) had a significantly
greater fall than the control group. This trial
suggests, not only the valuable opportunities that
may be available in industry for promoting health,
but that methods not involving long term medication
may be useful in controlling chronic disease.

Clearly these innovative approaches appear
attractive, but will they be effective in the day to
day routine of primary care – where most of this
responsibility must lie? Whitfield (52) has
suggested that there is a need for an interdisciplinary team for health education in primary
care and Tyser (86) feels that close links should be
established between the general practitioner and the
health education officer. The whole subject of what
is meant by community care must be explored – who is
expected to share the burden – family, friends, self-
help groups, volunteers or professionals. The
increasing burden of chronic disease presents a
challenge to all who are concerned to seek to improve
the quality of life of such patients.

SELF-HELP GROUPS

It is impossible to do more than refer very briefly
to the educational activities of self-help organizations – these being as diverse as the
organizations themselves.

One useful approach has been the establishment
of a self-help clearing house. In Britain this has
resulted in the production of 'Spotlight' – the
newsletter of the self-help clearing house and the
'Self-Help Reporter' in the United States. They
carry up-to-date information on new groups, change of
address, developments, current topics, new books,

conferences, meetings, etc. Because of the changing nature of self-help groups, this provision of up-to-date information is an essential reference to those who may be involved in advising those with problems so that they may obtain the benefit of the specific information and support available from a group.

Detailed information is supplied by organizations directly to their members. Some groups such as the Friedreich's Ataxia Group and the Psoriasis Association produce high quality newsletters 'FAX' and 'Beyond the Ointment' -covering activities at regional and national levels, meetings, individual achievements, up-to-date medical information, practical advice, holidays, competitions, encouragement, products, advice, letters, etc. Other groups concentrate on providing more technical advice which would otherwise be difficult for an individual to obtain. The Coeliac Society, through co-operation with manufacturers, provides up-to-date lists of food and products which are suitable for those who are allergic to gluten in cereals. They also list hotels prepared to cater for special diet, arrangements with airlines and explanatory sheets for use in foreign countries.

There may also be an educational effort aimed at a wider audience. A film such as 'Living with Pain', made by the Rheumatism and Arthritis Association, is primarily designed to encourage support for the Association. However, other films and books may be designed to inform the public generally or to provide specific information for relatives and friends who may care for the disabled person.

'Helping Hand', one of a series of television programmes on disablement, conveys the problem of getting about town, the daily aspects of living with handicap and the effects of paraplegia on marriage.

Another important component of many self-help groups is informing the professionals what self-help groups can do for their members. This is usually done at local level, by encouraging contact with relevant professionals and hospitals, but members of organizations can make a valuable contribution in undergraduate and postgraduate education of doctors, nurses, social workers and related health professionals.

An insight into what disease means to an individual can be enlightening to professionals who rarely are privileged to see the whole impact of illness on an individual or family. Professional journals sometimes publish articles by patients - some of whom are also professionals and this can be a useful education for professionals. Extracts from one such article are quoted below:

> I wish with all my heart and soul that I had not written this paper; for then I should still be where I spent five years' training to be, and where I planned to spend these years of my life, at work as a civil engineer, looking forward to coming home and playing football with my son. It would also mean, of course, that I would not have had to endure this agonising and devastating illness, motor neurone disease.
>
> A second point I want to emphasise early on is that I now spend my time in the wheelchair – I, who have fallen down so many times that I've forgotten (and that is <u>not</u> supposed to be a pun). I have fallen down in every room in my house: in the bathroom, the bedroom, the kitchen, the dining room, the lavatory, down the stairs and up the stairs. Every time, it is I who has had to get up and carry on. And I have to rely on somebody to wash me, dress me, take me to the lavatory, and to do even the most meaningless task for me – blow my nose or scratch my ear if it itches. I cannot do even a simple thing like wear a watch. So do not believe you understand – any more than I can understand what it is like to be blind: imagine, yes, but only for a few minutes at a time.
>
> The illness has continuously and relentlessly hammered me into the ground over the past four years, without ceasing. Now I have become what I consider doctors are to me in their professional capacity: neither use nor ornament. All the drugs, creams, and lotions that are used for my illness I could buy for myself over the chemist's counter, or find a substitute for at the off-licence.
>
> More important, there are only two people in the world who know how to look after me to my satisfaction and comfort: one is me and the other is my wife. Families know more about the illness and caring for the patient than any professional.
>
> In conclusion, I should like to draw attention to the following points. Firstly, the medical profession fails to understand the ordeal a person can go through not only while he is in a wheelchair but, more significantly, while he is still trying to stay on his feet. Secondly, preparing this paper has not made any

difference to my condition. Thirdly, how do you explain to the public what this disease is? People cannot respond to the fact that I have motor neurone disease as they could if it were multiple sclerosis or Parkinson's disease, of which they have a vague understanding or awareness. Because of this problem a leaflet was printed to make the general public more aware of the disease. It may not be perfect, but anyone who can write a better one for us is welcome to do so. Fourthly, and to his eternal credit, my G.P. has never stopped coming to see me, no matter what the circumstances, even though he can do nothing constructive (but neither can anyone else).

Such articles may encourage humility in professionals and make them realize the breadth of support that is required and the contribution made by families, friends, support groups and self-help groups. Lists of organizations have been published by the Sunday Times and the Kings Fund. (88)

GENERAL MEDIA

The range of books available to patients and their relatives or helpers is very similar to that described in the last chapter. It includes books by professionals which provide broadly based current medical information, and are like simplified text books, publications for groups or individuals who have personal experience and highlight the care, supporting and encouraging aspects of self-care, and thirdly, publications from a particular standpoint who believe that one approach will lead to the cure or amelioration of the condition.

A review of the British Medical Journal (89) commenced with the comment - 'Hooray - more work for patients'. This humorous comment indicates the enormous increase in the number and diversity of books which are available on specific illnesses or problems - whether it is a disease, a medical condition, a time of life or a sexual problem, there are a multitude of books on the shelves of the bookshops. Presumably their existence is a testimony to their purchase and perhaps their use.

Family doctor booklets are an example of an officially approved publication from the British Medical Association. These have been going for many years and now come in a wide range of topics.

Another series produced by Oxford University Press includes: 'Migraine: the Facts', (90) and 'Asthma: the Facts', (91) which again provide simple well-balanced authoritative information.

From one of the long established and successful self-help groups a book has been produced which brings together the distillation of years of experience of coping with a problem that is not well catered for by medical treatment alone. The very title of the book - 'Cystitis - a complete self-help guide' (92) is indicative of the comprehensive approach by Angela Kilmartin whose name is almost synonymous with the society.

The International Year of Disabled People provided an opportunity for new interest, new programmes and new publications. Dr Wendy Greengross summed up some of the activities in an article in the British Medical Journal - 'Medicine and the Media': (93)

> There are a plethora of attitudes to disablement ranging from genuine concern and caring through a feeling that 'they' ought to be grateful for everything and anything they get to a belief that the disabled should be the responsibility of the State, or the social services, or their friends and family. One of the aims of the International Year of Disabled People (IYDP) is to encourage a questioning of assumptions, so that eventually disabled people will be given the services and care that <u>they</u> need rather than the services and care the <u>able-bodied</u> need or want to give.
>
> The media have accepted their role in this with enthusiasm and alacrity, examining the needs of disabled people and generally bringing them out of the closet and forcing upon viewers and listeners some realisation that there are many severley disabled people around who are capable of speaking for themselves as intelligently, as movingly, and as wittily as anyone else, and that inside twisted, even grotesque, bodies there are ordinary people who are as nice or nasty as anyone else. Quite a change from a few years ago when the editor of a well-known women's magazine refused a series on the emotional problems of the disabled, saying with some distaste, 'My readers don't want to know anything about that'.
>
> She also quotes 'That's Life' which put Paul

Heiney into a wheelchair for a week. This brought
home to viewers the subjective experience of the
wheel-chair bound: no ramps onto the pavemnents, an
endless trail to find a 'disabled lavatory' which was
in vain, since it had been closed because of cutbacks. Heiney also complained that once in a
wheelchair he became, "a non-person, disregarded and
ignored by those around him". (93)

Dr Greengross mentions other programmes such as
'Woman's Hour', 'You and Yours' and 'Does he Take
Sugar', all of which have given insights into the way
disabled people are treated.

It is those programmes made by disabled people,
such as Joan Shenton's 'Help' and the Graeae Theatre
Company 'Getting away from Sidney' however, which
confront us most bluntly with our own responses to
disablement and give us, Dr. Greengross says, the
opportunity to "join in the laughter with them as
equals, without embarrassment". (93)

Source books of organizations, aids, techniques, services and rights form a significant part of
the general books. (94) There are also specialised
books such as 'Help Yourselves: a handbook for
hemiplegics and their families' (95) which covers
subjects such as independence, mobility, personal
hygiene, dressing, at the table, in the kitchen,
housework, the weekly wash, work and other
activities, speech problems, problems of perception
and changed personality, sexual problems and outside
help. It is also important to remember that
organizations not related to health may produce
specific publications such as, 'London - A Guide for
Disabled Visitors' by the Tourist Board. (96)

The experiences of a family with a problem, such
as a handicapped child, can provide encouragement to
others in similar situations. 'Kith and Kids' (97)
shows how one family fought for the best of their
handicapped child - comprehensive assessment and
special schooling - and how with first one and then
several other families they set up Kith and Kids
which met on Sundays mainly to overcome the
loneliness that affected all of them, and grew into a
structured programme of activities and training for
the children, and informal support for the families.

Practical advice in an eminently readable form
is the main attribute of 'A Patient's Guide to
Operations'. (98) It would be extremely interesting
to examine the value of books such as this in
allaying anxiety, providing information on hospital
procedures and on the value of the practical advice
on recovery and activities such as driving cars and

return to work.

The alternative approaches tend to emphasize what individuals can achieve through their own action to solve their problem – by diet, change of lifestyle or natural remedies. 'How to Lift Your Depression' (99) is based on elementary behaviour theory and focusses on the individual's capacity to gain control over the environment and on his or her response to it. 'Nature Cure for Sinusitis' (100) (one of a series which includes arthritis, asthma, skin troubles and varicose veins) emphasizes treatment by natural means and what be achieved without drugs, which in the authors opinion merely suppress symptoms. True health is seen as related to what people eat, drink and breathe and that prevention by natural means is better than supression through medication.

The wealth of material now being published is an indication of the immense interest being shown by the public in health issues. The value and use of such material has not been evaluated and its use by public and professionals is not understood. It is not known whether it fosters communcation between doctors and patients, or whether it reduces it. Studies examining the links between information and participation and studies of the potential value of educational material in hospitals, health centres, waiting rooms and informal groups are urgently required.

TABLE 11.1 Guide to minimum information needed to enable patients to make treatment with a prescribed drug effective and safe

1. To know how to take the drug:	1.1	To take a specific dose	1.1.1 Amount of drug per tablet or other dosage form
			1.1.2 Average dose and dose range, adult
			1.1.3 Average dose and dose range, child
	1.2	To take a dose in a specific manner	1.2.1 Manner directed by dosage form or drug
	1.3	To take a dose at specific times	1.3.1 Clock time
			1.3.2 Time since last dose
			1.3.3 Time since or until food intake
			1.3.4 Duration of treatment
2. To know how to store the drug:	2.1	To store it properly	2.1.1 Storage conditions
	2.2.	To recognise the time at which the medicine becomes subpotent	2.2.2 Expiry date
			2.2.3 Event showing deterioration
3. To know how the drug is expected to help:	3.1	To recall the basic facts about the complaint	3.1.1 Disease or symptoms to be affected
			3.1.2 Potential consequence of compliance
			3.1.3 Potential consequence of non-compliance
			3.2.1 Events showing effect
	3.2	To recognise the desired effect and act upon its absence	3.2.2 Time at which to expect effect
			3.2.3 Direction for follow-up if there is no effect
4. To know how to recognise problems caused by the drug:	4.1	To recognise unwanted effects and act if they occur	4.1.1 Events showing unwanted effect
			4.1.2 Direction for follow-up of events
	4.2	To recall that certain unwanted effects can only be detected by clinical examination or tests	4.2.1 Unwanted effects that the patient cannot observe
			4.2.2 Direction for detection of such effects
	4.3	To recall circumstances indicating need for change of treatment, and act if they occur	4.3.1 Change in the patient's state
			4.3.2 Direction for follow-up of change
			4.3.3 Other drug added to therapy
			4.3.4 Direction for follow-up of drug addiction
	4.4	To verify components of medicine	4.4.1 Name of drug and "active" excipient
			4.4.2 Direction for follow-up of "action"
	4.5	To act if overdosage occurs	4.5.1 Direction for follow-up of occurrence

FIGURE 11.1 Supplementary Information on Medication Card

TETRACYCLINE
Supplementary Information on Medication

Rx# _____

Pharmacist _____

Tetracycline is used to treat or prevent infection.

Effects on normal activities:

Sometimes, while you are taking tetracycline and for some time after, it can make the skin more sensitive to sun or to sunlamps - you could get a severe sunburn. If your skin becomes sensitive, tell your doctor, wear protective clothing, sunglasses. Ask your pharmacist about sunscreens. Some types of tetracycline can cause lightheadednesses, dizziness, loss of balance or fainting. Do not drive or operate dangerous machinery.

When you take your tetracycline:

Take your medicine **exactly** as directed on the prescription label. Some tetracyclines are made to be taken without food, with a full glass of water, about 1 hour before or 2 hours after eating. Your doctor or pharmacist will tell you if you have received this type. Doses should be evenly spaced, during the waking hours.

Liquid tetracycline should be WELL SHAKEN before each dose.

Finish ALL your medication unless the doctor tells you to stop or else your infection might come back.

Stomach upset, vomiting, loss of appetite may occur. If stomach upset does occur, try taking doses with some crackers or a light snack. This effect may disappear as you get used to this drug. **Mild** diarrhea may also occur. If these effects get worse, call your doctor.

If you FORGET a dose:

Take your medicine as soon as you realize that you have missed a dose. Then take your medicine at the same time as before.

What else may happen?

While taking this medication you should watch for any unwanted effects. The following signs are not common, but if they do happen, call your doctor immediately. He will tell you if you should still take this drug.

- rash, hives, itching
- rectal itch or (in women) vaginal itch or unusual discharge

ALWAYS REMEMBER:
- Tell your doctor and pharmacist what other drugs you are taking
- Tell any new doctor or dentist that you visit that you are taking tetracycline
- Certain things may interfere with tetracycline:
    - milk, dairy products - such as cheese, ice cream, cottage cheese
    - antacid (stomach) preparations, sodium bicarbonate (baking soda)
    - iron and some vitamins.

    Do not take these for 2-3 hours **before** or at least 2 hours **after** you take tetracycline. The pharmacist can advise you about these products.
- Some liquid tetracycline contain sugar. Diabetics should check with the pharmacist or doctor for advice.
- If the doctor has told you to stop taking tetracycline flush any unused drug down the toilet. OUTDATED TETRACYCLINE CAN BE HARMFUL.

If you need more information, ask your doctor or pharmacist.

Developed by the Canadian Pharmaceutical Association in co-operation with the Health Protection Branch, Health & Welfare Canada, the medical profession and medication users.

April, 1980.

Patient Education

FIGURE 11.2 Supplementary Information on Medication Card

ANTICOAGULANT DRUGS
Supplementary Information on Medication

Rx# _____

Pharmacist _____

This drug is sometimes called a "blood thinner". It is used to stop you from getting blood clots.

If you are taking the anticoagulant called "phenindione" your urine may become reddish-orange coloured. Do not worry. This effect is normal and harmless.

Effects on normal activities:

Anticoagulants make you bleed more easily, so you should use a soft toothbrush and an electric razor for shaving. Do not do things where you could easily get hurt such as soccer, tackle football, horseback riding.

ALWAYS carry a card which says that you take this drug and what your blood type is. If you are going to take this drug for more than 3 months, you should get a medication alert bracelet or necklace.

When you take anticoagulants:

Take your medicine exactly as ordered on the prescription label. Take each day's dose at the same time of day. Never take more or less medication per day than your doctor has ordered.

Other drugs can change the action of anticoagulants. While you are taking this drug do not stop, start or change the amount of other drugs you are also taking. Ask your doctor first.

For colds, headaches, arthritis, or other types of pain DO NOT TAKE **ANY** MEDICINE CONTAINING ASA (Asprin). ASA when taken with anticoagulants could cause you to bleed. Ask your doctor or pharmacist to suggest a different product to treat these conditions.

If you FORGET a dose:

Take your medicine as soon as you realize that you have missed a dose. If you do not remember until the next day, take only ONE dose. DO NOT take a double dose. If you forget two days in a row, or twice in one week, call your doctor.

What else may happen?

While you are taking this medication, you should watch for any unwanted effects. The following signs are not common but if they do happen, call your doctor immediately. He will tell you if you should still take this drug.
- pink or brown urine
- black or red bowel movements
- nose bleeds
- numerous large bruises
- swelling in a joint (such as knee, ankle, elbow, wrist)
- reddish brown vomit or saliva
- different or very heavy bleeding during your period
- severe back pain

If you cannot reach your doctor, call a hospital emergency department for advice.

ALWAYS REMEMBER
- Tell any other doctor, dentist or pharmacist you see that you are taking this drug.
- Contact your doctor right away if you become sick with the flu, or get a fever, vomiting or diarrhea
- The action of this drug is easily changed by other drugs. Do not take any non-prescription drugs without asking your pharmacist first. Even before buying **vitamins** or **mineral oil,** tell the pharmacist you are taking this anticoagulant drug.
- Avoid alcohol. Do not have more than 1 alcoholic drink a day. A regular balanced diet is important. If you plan to change your eating habits for any reason, check with your doctor first.

If you need more information, ask your doctor or pharmacist.

Developed by the Canadian Pharmaceutical Association in co-operation with the Health Protection Branch, Health & Welfare Canada, the medical profession and medication users. April, 1980.

205

TABLE 11.2 MEDICINES IN THE HOME

Who or what first gave adults the idea of using
the non-prescribed medicines they had taken

Who or what first gave the idea:	%
Spouse	7
Parents/grandparents	18
Other relatives	5
Friends, etc.	13
Doctor	10
Para-medical people	4
Chemist	6
Advertising	8
Can't remember etc.	22
Other, including reading	7
Number of medicines (=100%)	1,902

From: Dunnell & Cartwright, 1972

NOTES

1.   Annas GJ. The Rights of Hospital Patients New York: Avon Books, 1975, pp.25-27.

2.   Boyle CM. Differences Between Patients' and Doctors' Interpretation of some Common Medical Terms. British Medical Journal 1970; 2: 286-289.

3.   Cartwright A. Human Relations and Hospital Care London: Routledge and Kegan Paul, 1964.

4.   Dunn K. Planning for Patient Education in General Practice: Patient Knowledge of Specified Conditions in General Practice University of Nottingham: M.Med.Sci. Thesis, 1978.

5.   Coutts L. Health Teaching in Nursing: An Exploratory Study University of Nottingham: M.Med.Sci. Thesis, 1979.

6.   Dunkelman H. Patient's knowledge of Their Condition and Treatment - How it Might be Improved. British Medical Journal 1979; 2: 311-314.

7.   Pratt L., Seligman A. and Reader G. Physician Views on the Level of Medical Information among Patients. American Journal of Public Health 1957; 47: 1277-1283.

8.   Cartwright A. and Anderson R. Patients and Their Doctors 1977. Journal of the Royal College of General Practitioners 1980; Occasional Paper 8.

9.   Byrne PS. and Long BEL. Doctors Talking to Patients London: H.M.S.O., 1976.

10. Fletcher C. Listening and Talking to Patients, I-IV. British Medical Journal 1980; 281: 845-847, 931-933, 994-996, 1056-1058.

11. Davis Lord Justice Edmund. The Patient's Right to Know the Truth. Proceedings of the Royal Society of Medicine 1973; 66: 533-538.

12. Porter AMW. Drug Defaulting in a General Practice. British Medical Journal 1969; 1: 218-227

13. Blackwell B. Drug Therapy Patient Compliance. New England Journal of Medicine 1973; 289: 249.

14. Eaton G. Non-compliance. In Mapes R. (Ed.) Prescribing Practice and Drug Usage London: Croom Helm, 1980.

15. Haynes RB., Taylor DW. and Sackett DL. (Eds.) Compliance in Health Care Baltimore: The John Hopkins University Press, 1979.

16. Stimson GV. Obeying Doctor's Orders: A View from the Other Side. Social Science and Medicine 1976; 8: 97-104.

17. Vaisrub G. You Can Lead a Horse to Water ... Journal of the American Medical Association 1975; 234: 80-81.

18. Leading Article. Non-compliance: Does it

matter? British Medical Journal 1979; 2: 1168.

19. Sheps SC. and Kirkpatrick RA. Hypertension. Mayo Clinic Proceedings 1975; 50: 709-720.

20. Faunch R. What the Public Wants to Know. Letter. British Medical Journal 1979; 1: 1627.

21. Parkin DM., Henney CR., Quirk J. and Crooks. Deviation from Prescribed Drug Treatment After Discharge from Hospital. British Medical Journal 1976; 2: 686-688.

22. Downie WW., Leatham PA., Rhind VM. and Wright V. Steroid Cards: Patient Compliance. British Medical Journal 1977; 1: 428.

23. Ezedum S. and Kerr DNG. Collaborative Care of Hypertensives Using a Shared Record. British Medical Journal 1977; 2: 1402-1403.

24. Everett CR. Repeat Prescription Cards. Practitioner 1974; 213: 707-711.

25. Baxendale C., Gourlay M. and Gibson JM. A Self-medication Retraining Programme. British Medical Journal 1978; 2: 1278-1279.

26. Wandless I. and Davie JW. Can Drug Compliance in the Elderly be Improved? British Medical Journal 1977; 1: 359-361.

27. MacDonald ET., MacDonald JB. and Phoenix M. Improving Drug Compliance After Hospital Discharge. British Medical Journal 1977; 2: 618-621.

28. Tulloch AJ. Repeat Prescribing for Elderly Patients. British Medical Journal 1981; 282: 1672-1675.

29. Martys CR. Adverse Drug Reaction to Drugs in General Practice. British Medical Journal 1979; 2: 1194-1197.

30. Leading Article. Drug Information for Patients: Keep it Simple. British Medical Journal 1980; 281: 1393.

31. Herxheimer A. and Lionel WDW. Minimum Information Needed by Prescribers. British Medical Journal 1978; 2: 1128-1132.

32. Hermann F., Herxheimer A. and Lionel NDW. Package Inserts for Prescribed Medicines. What Minimum Information do Patients Need? British Medical Journal 1978; 2: 1132-1135.

33. Leading Article. Patient Package Inserts. British Medical Journal 1978; 2: 586.

34. Honey E. Medicine and the Media. British Medical Journal 1980; 281: 674-675.

35. Weibert RT. and Dee DA. Experience in an Organized Patient Education Program. Journal of the American Pharmaceutical Association 1976; 16: 450-452.

36. Canadian Pharmaceutical Association.

Supplementary Information on Medication. In association with the Health Protection Branch, Health and Welfare, Canada, the medical profession, and medication users. Canada: Canadian Pharmaceutical Association, 1980.

37. Fink JL. Self-medication. American Journal of Pharmacy 1976; 148: 90-96.

38. Shulman S. and Shulman J. Operating a Two Card Medication Record System in General Practice Pharmacy. Practitioner 1980; 224: 989-992.

39. Ettlinger PRA. and Freeman GK. General Practice Compliance Study: Is it Worth being a Personal Doctor? British Medical Journal 1981; 282: 1192-1194.

40. Sehnert KW. How to be your own Doctor - Sometimes New York: Grossett and Dunlap, 1975.

41. Vickery DW. and Fries JF. Take Care of Yourself. A Consumer's Guide to Medical Care Massachusetts: Addison-Wesley, 1976.

42. Anderson JAD. (Ed.) Self-medication Lancaster: M.T.P. Press, 1979.

43. Cust G. and Wells JP. Home Medicines - Communication, Advertising and Education. In Anderson JAD. (Ed.) Self-medication Lancaster: M.T.P. Press, 1979.

44. Eliott-Binns CP. An Analysis of Lay-Medicine. Journal of the Royal College of General Practitioners 1973; 23: 255-264.

45. Dunnell K. and Cartwright A. Medicine Takers, Prescribers and Hoarders London: Routledge and Kegan Paul, 1972.

46. Braithwaite A. and Cooper P. Analgesic Effects of Branding in Treatment of Headaches. British Medical Journal 1981; 282: 1576-1578.

47. Lawrence DR. and Black JW. The Medicine you Take London: Fontana Books, 1978.

48. Parish P. Medicines: A Guide for Everybody Harmondsworth: Penguin, 1976.

49. Health Education Council. Treating Yourself - A Guide to Self-medication London: H.E.C., 1975.

50. Scottish Health Education Unit. Help Yourself to Health Edinburgh: S.H.E.U., 1978.

51. Humphreys L. Self Responsibility in Health Care. An Evaluation of the Health Education Council's Booklet 'Treating Yourself' Reading University: M.A. Dissertation, 1976.

52. Whitfield M. Group Health Education in General Practice. Journal of the Royal College of General Practitioners 1976; 24: 529-536.

53. Gaskell PC. and Watson LM. Trial of a Self-

help Scheme. Update 1978; 17: 661-667.

54. Morrell DC., Avery AJ. and Watking CJ. Management of Minor Illness. British Medical Journal 1980; 281: 769-771.

55. Anderson JE., Morrell DC., Avery AJ. and Watkins CJ. Evaluation of A Patient Education Manual. British Medical Journal 1980; 281: 924-926.

56. Section of General Practice. A Doctor's Responsibility to Society. Proceedings of the Royal Society of Medicine 1977; 70: 21-23.

57. Whitfield M. The Pharmacist's Contribution to Medical Care. The Practitioner 1968; 200: 434-438.

58. Webb B. The Retail Pharmacist and Drug Treatment. Journal of the Royal College of General Practitioners 1976; 26: Supplement No. 1: 81-85.

59. Harris J. To Investigate the Determinants of the Advisory and Information Service and the Potential for Health Education in Retail Pharmacy University of Nottingham, M.Med.Sci. Thesis, 1980.

60. Eardley A., Davis F. and Wakefield J. Health Education by Chance: The Unmet Needs of Patients in Hospital and After. International Journal of Health Education 1975; 18: 19-23.

61. Hobbs P., Eardley A. and Thornton M. Health Education with Patients in Hospital. The Health Education Journal 1977; 36: 35-41.

62. Richards RF. and Kalmer H. (Eds.) Patient Education. Health Education Monographs 1974; 2: 1-92.

63. Valiga TM. (Issue Editor) Education for Self-care. Topics in Clinical Nursing 1980; 2: (entire issue).

64. Baranovsky LV. and Jurieva KA. Developing a Model for Health Education. Intervention in the Hospital Setting. International Journal of Health Education 1981; 18: 19-23.

65. Gay P. and Pitkeathley J. When I went Home ... A Study of Patients Discharged from Hospital London: King Edwards Fund for London, 1979.

66. Davis MZ. The Organizational, International and Care Oriented Conditions for Patient Participation in Continuity of Care. A Framework for Staff Intervention. Social Science and Medicine 1980; 14A: 39-49.

67. Ellis DA., Hopkin JM. Leitch AG. and Crofton Sir John. "Doctor's Orders" Controlled Trial of Supplementary Written Information for Patients. British Medical Journal 1979; 1: 456.

68. O'Hanrahan M., O'Malley K. and O'Brien ET. Printed Information for the Lay Public on Cardio-vascular Disease. British Medical Journal 1980; 281:

597-599.

69. Breckenridge A. Self-monitoring - A Symposium. Chairman's introduction. Prescribers Journal 1976; 16: 26-39 (complete symposium).

70. Sonksew PH., Judd SL. and Lowy C. Home Monitoring of Blood Glucose. Lancet 1978; 1: 729-732.

71. Walford S., Gale EAM., Allison SP. and Tattersall RB. Self-monitoring of Blood Glucose. Lancet 1978; 1: 732-735.

72. Steel JM., Cramb R. and Duncan LJP. How Useful are Patient-operated Blood Glucose Meters? Practitioner 1980; 224: 651-653.

73. Peacock I., Hunter JC., Walford S., Allison SP., Davison J., Clarke P., Symonds EM. and Tattersall RB. Self-monitoring of Blood Glucose in Diabetic Pregnancy. British Medical Journal 1979; 2: 1333-1336.

74. Davenport RR., Ferguson DE., Fitzpatrick EO, and White BW. Dieticians, Nurses Teach Diabetic Patients. Hospitals 1974; 48: 81-82.

75. Duncan JG. Teaching Commonsense Health Care Habits to Diabetic Patients. Geriatrics 1976; 31: 93-96.

76. Worth C. Foot Problems in Diabetic Patients: An Analysis of Hospital Records and Follow up of Selected Patients University of Nottingham, B.Med.Sci. Dissertation, 1981.

77. Delbridge L. Educational and Psychological Factors in the Management of Diabetes in Childhood. Medical Journal of Australia 1975; 2: 737-739.

78. Stokes JB., Payne GH. and Cooper T. Hypertension Control - The Challenge of Patient Education. New England Journal of Medicine 1973; 289: 1369-1370.

79. Wilkinson PR. and Rafferty EB. Patient's Attitude to Measuring their own Blood Pressure. British Medical Journal 1978; 1: 824.

80. Green LW., Levine DM. and Deeds S. Clinical Trial of Health Education for Hypertensive Outpatients. Design and Baseline Data. Preventive Medicine 1975; 4: 417-425.

81. Spiegel AD. Patient and Physician Education. Medical Care 1965; 3: 46-52.

82. Coope JR. Management of Hypertension in General Practice. A.B.C. of Blood Pressure Management. British Medical Journal 1981; 282: 1380-1382.

83. Laher M., O'Malley K., O'Brien E., O'Hanrahan M. and O'Boyle C. Educational Value of Printed Information for Patients with Hypertension. British Medical Journal 1981; 282: 1360-1361.

84. Tilson E. Organization for Long-term Management of Hypertension: The Trade Union as a Compliance Mechanism in the Treatment of Hypertension. Bulletin of New York Academy of Medicine 1976; 52: 714-717.

85. Patel C., Marmot MG. and Terry DJ. Controlled Trial of Biofeedback Aided Behavioural Methods in Reducing Mild Hypertension. British Medical Journal 1981; 282: 2005-2007.

86. Tyser PA. Health Education in General Practice. Community Health 1975; 4: 179-184.

87. Carus R. Motor Neurone Disease: A Demeaning Illness. British Medical Journal 1980; 281: 455-456.

88. Sayer K. (Compiler) King's Fund Directory of Organizations for Patients and Disabled People London: Pitman Medical, 1979.

89. Last P. Book review. British Medical Journal 1979; 1: 1786.

90. Rose EC. Migraine: The Facts Oxford: Oxford University Press, 1979.

91. Lane D. and Storr A. Asthma: The Facts Oxford: Oxford University Press, 1979.

92. Kilmartin A. Cystitis: A Complete Self-help Guide London: Hamlyn, 1980.

93. Medicine and the Media. British Medical Journal 1981; 282: 391.

94. Hale G. (Ed.) The Source Book for the Disabled: An Illustrated Guide to Easier More Independent Living for Physically Disabled People, Their Families and Friends London: Paddington Press, 1979.

95. Jay P. Help Yourselves. A Handbook for Hemiplegics and Their Families Hornchurch: Ian Henry Publications, 1979.

96. London Tourist Board. London - A Guide for Disabled Visitors London: London Tourist Board, 26 Grosvenor Gardens, London, 1981.

97. Collins M. and Collins D. Kith and Kids - Self-Help for Families of the Handicapped London: Souvenir Press, 1976.

98. Delvin D. A Patient's Guide to Operations Harmondsworth: Penguin, 1981.

99. Juniper D. How to Lift Your Depression London: Open Books, 1978.

100. Quick C. Nature Cure for Sinusitis Wellingborough: Thorsons Publishers Ltd., 1974.

Chapter Twelve

CHANGING PROFESSIONAL ROLES AND THE WIDER SCENE

Neither in principle nor in practice can we expect
patients to be accorded respect and responsibilities
if the same process is not going on in inter-profess-
ional relationships. Participation applies not only
to doctor and patient but also to the varying members
of any particular health team and to the relationship
with the wider group of professionals and non-
professionals who may be involved in many health
issues. Participation is unlikely to thrive in an
atmosphere which is autocratic or bureaucratic and
where people with differing skills and experience are
not accorded respect, and their potential
contribution recognized.
    Task demarcation and its concomitant unequal
distribution of wealth and status is to some extent
based on tradition and mystique. From the discussion
in earlier sections in this book it is apparent that
a re-appraisal of the functions of the various health
workers is required. There are signs that this is now
taking place - sometimes this is initiated from
within a health service or professional group while
in other instances it results from community concern
and a recognition of unmet need. This chapter will
examine some of the groups that are currently
considering change and some of the situations which
are being reappraised.

A REORIENTATION

This recognition that a change in directiion in
health care is required has been greatly stimulated
by the activities of the World Health Organization.
A recent article by Dr Halfdan Mahler, Director
General, World Health Organization, entitled "World
Health is Indivisible", (1) puts the new approach

very clearly.

> If social and economic factors, including the
> influence of the environment and individual and
> community life styles are responsible for most
> ill health, wisdom demands that we deal first
> and foremost with these factors. Therefore,
> technical policy must respond to social policy
> rather than to the search for technical
> perfection. All the medical techniques, the
> plethora of equipment and drugs, the
> complicated facilities, the labyrinth of
> logistical support and the hordes of supporting
> staff would be justified if they were effective,
> but the effectiveness of much of them remains
> unproved. I am not doubting the sincerity of
> those who apply the ever-growing range of health
> technologies at ever-increasing costs to
> society. But I am challenging them to re-assess
> the usefulness of these methods and to reflect
> on their cost and on society's ability to pay
> for them.
> Wisdom also demands that health measures
> be applied where they are most needed, most
> effective and least costly. This is the
> rationale for the growing insistence on the
> delivery of primary health care. It is also the
> rationale for organizing the other levels of the
> health system to support and manage primary
> health care.

Emphasis is clearly laid on the influence of
environmental factors in health and on the importance
of primary care, particularly in the developing
countries. This latter has been influential in
looking at new ways of tackling health needs, the
development of new categories of health workers and
appropriate use of technology.

A NEW CONCEPT OF PRIMARY CARE
– NEW CATEGORIES OF HEALTH WORKERS

In the western countries, despite the differences in
health care systems, there is a general expectation
that medical care from doctors is available and
fairly easily accessible to all who require it. This
however is by no means true of many developing
countries where doctors are few and where access to
any health worker, traditional healer or religious
healer may be difficult. From the need to meet this

enormous gap in service provision has resulted some
of the more imaginative innovations and changes in
policy. These have implications not only for the
developing countries but also for the developed. The
World Health Organization has set the target of
"Health for All by the Year 2000". Integral to this
approach has been the development of some form of
primary care health worker whose functions are
clearly related to a particular community's needs. As
Mahler again states: (2)

> The Member States of the World Health
> Organization have committed themselves to the
> decisive socio-economic task of providing
> health for all by the year 2000. This cannot be
> achieved through the conventional health
> service development of the past few decades.
> Primary health care is a new concept which
> demands action at the social periphery, where
> the old order rarely penetrated. The health
> auxilliary will play a vital role in this re-
> orientation of health services towards
> increased social relevance.

The key role of auxilliary workers is further
described by Katherine Elliott: (3)

> Primary health care begins with human beings,
> families, homes and communities and cannot be
> separated out from general social and economic
> improvement. Everyone must have access to
> primary health care, find its form and its costs
> acceptable, and be willing to participate
> appropriately. To meet complex health needs,
> referral routes to specialist medical services
> must be provided and safe-guarded. Auxilliary
> workers can nevertheless carry most of the
> primary health care burden because experience
> has shown that primary health care services work
> most satisfactorily when they make use of local
> people, who remain part of the communities they
> serve but who have been given the right kind of
> technical and social training to enable them to
> respond effectively to local needs. They then
> become an invaluable resource for the new style
> of health services which are required to meet
> the target set by the World Health Organization
> of health for all by the year 2000.
> In most countries now health services are
> being reshaped with greater flexibility in
> mind. New ways are being sought and found to

train and to integrate increasing numbers of
auxilliary health workers in systems which
inevitably vary by country and by community
according to the needs to be met and the human
and material resources available for this
purpose. Much more is being recorded about the
different approaches being tried and attempts
have been made to evaluate some of them.

In several developing countries experimental
schemes have been established which are broadly
similar in that they aim to provide a pyramidial
system of health care, from a community or primary
health care worker, sometimes illiterate, drawn from
a village and given medical training, through an
intermediate local worker, to a centre staffed by
doctors and ultimately to a specialized hospital.
The exact nature of the structure varies from one
country to another. Not only are there experiments in
the structure of the services provided, but the
training of these workers, the tools they use, their
origins and their supervision have all been the
subject of trial. Katherine Elliott's book provides
reference to all these aspects.

Tanzania was one of the first countries to build
a health care system on this basis. An article in the
Lancet (4) described the reasons for this innovative
approach in that country, while more recent
descriptions have outlined the measures adopted and
the ways in which they have developed over the years.
(5,6) Another country, known to one of the authors,
where there are problems in providing services over
enormous areas with relatively few staff and
resources is Sudan, (7) where considerable emphasis
has been laid on the training of health workers who
will combine preventive and curative skills at the
village level. Indeed a special category of worker
has been designated for the Nomadic population in
Sudan. There is a suggestion that in countries where
there is a large number of doctors, albeit not evenly
distributed, that the use of such auxilliaries has
been less successful. Again, based on one of the
author's discussions during a visit to Pakistan, this
would seem to be true of the Health Guards Programme
in that country. A further development in Pakistan
has been employing a husband and wife team as the
community health worker to promote a joint approach
to family health care.

A thorough account and an evaluation study of
training programmes has been carried out in Iran. (8)
In the various different programmes a variety of

manuals, handbooks and flow charts (9,10,11) for the health workers have been designed and evaluated. The World Health Organization has played a key role in promoting such programmes and aiding in the educational process: (12) the most recent development seeks to promote communication, exchange of ideas and co-ordination between centres with the establishment of a bank of educational materials.

Bennett (13) in a recent article, examines some of the issues which have resulted from this movement and how these are likely to affect future planning. He reviews some of the points made by other writers on this subject and although it is not possible here to examine them all in depth, it may be useful to list some of them to stimulate continuing debate and discussion.

- only in countries in which there has been a fundamental shift of wealth and power to those who previously had least and in which there has been an exercise of that power for the strengthening of equity and community is the model of primary care approached.
- the creation of barefoot doctors was a political act to change patterns of control over health care
- primary health care forms an integral part, both of the country's health system of which it is the central function and main focus of the overall social and economic development of the community.
- the term 'delivery of health services' is no longer strictly correct, as it implies something delivered to people from above or centrally, whereas the concept gaining acceptance is of health services generated within the periphery and linking up with a referral system. The focal point is thus the community and the perspective has been reversed being no longer the former one of viewing the high-cost technology teaching hospital as the centre of the medical universe.
- one of the mechanisms to stimulate community participation is 'self-diagnosis', a process of involvement of the community in surveying its own problem.

To some this is a fashionable bandwagon, political rhetoric, a new interest for international agencies and a threat to the established professions. To others it is seen as the only real hope of developing a health care system that can meet some of the needs of a large number of countries. Some of these countries have illustrated their belief by a financial commitment and sometimes a re-orientation in their administrative structure. In all there is a clear need to define priorities and to build an infrastructure for health related to the needs and demands of a community. (14)

Another area which has recently been the focus for review by the World Health Organization has been the role of the traditional healer. (15) Instead of seeking to prohibit the activities of the traditional healer or to reduce their opportunities for practice by means of comprehensive freely available orthodox practitioners, there is now a move to attempt to involve them as members of the team, to seek to make use of their skills and experience and their relationship with the community and at the same time to change practices and habits that are harmful to health. The traditional birth attendant in countries such as Sudan is one example of where this integration appears to be working well, but in Pakistan there has been the opposite result, with the alternative practitioners seeing this new approach as an encouragement to their already large and powerful organization and they are seeking to promote separate development. It is interesting to compare the "Granny midwife" (16) of twenty years ago in the southern parts of the United States with the current changes taking place in the developing countries – is there to be competition or integration? Will the traditional practitioner give way to the orthodox practitioners in the next generation? Will the skills and experience of the traditional practitioners be kept or submerged?

Some of the dilemmas have recently been summarized by Una Maclean in a review of the World Health Organization Report (17)

> It is clearly impossible, in the foreseeable future, to provide the mass of man- and womankind with conventional doctors. They must be treated by auxilliary health workers, or look to lay healers. Until recently the study of the nature and extent of the practice of indigenous healers has tended to be regarded as a purely academic exercise, the chosen domain of a small sub-group of anthropologists, whose findings could not conceivably be of concern to the main medical establishment of any country. Now W.H.O. is attempting to redress the balance.

The idea of involving traditional practitioners in health care seems admirable in
principle, but there are formidable methodological and political barriers to its implementation.

In the first place, traditional healers
deal with an exceedingly wide range of human
misfortunes and maladies. Whilst the sorting
system of local healers for any particular
society may well fit the cultural concepts of
their clientele they certainly do not match
conventional, Western diagnostic categories and
standards. Next, in the realm of practice, it
will be necessary to establish criteria for
sorting beneficient from harmful treatments, in
itself a daunting task. It will be necessary,
furthermore, to decide who are to be the
potential learners and to designate those who
are to provide their teaching or, rather, their
supplementary training, since they already
possess skills of their own. There is one
helpful model for this kind of exercise namely
the up-grading of traditional birth attendants.

The W.H.O. report declares that there is a
need for 'a clear definition of objectives' but
fails to provide such definitions. Instead it
has to fall back upon brief descriptions of
stated research priorities in Mexico and
Nigeria. There is only the scantiest reference
to the Chinese experience, but rather more space
is devoted to outlines of indigenous medicine in
Sri Lanka, Egypt, Ghana and India.

This is certainly a fascinating area for
exploration, relating as it does to differing
cultural ways of responding to the entire
spectrum of disease, disability and death. The
Western trained doctor or health planner,
concerned with rapid action, should set about a
strict sorting of the advantages and disadvantages of traditional and modern care
systems for different age groups, disease
states, places and peoples. Different
organizational structures will need to be
devised for widely varying political settings.

The topic positively bristles with
difficulties and challenges. How, for instance,
can one measure effectiveness? How will
established health professionals and governments react? But W.H.O.has made a worthwhile and
welcome start in publicizing a neglected area
and might with profit consider as well the

findings of established research in this field.

These changes are not limited to the developing world. As the nurse withdraws from her traditional role of doctor's help-mate, some commentators are seeing scope for a new type of health worker – the aide. It already happens of course in remote situations that nurses alone do the job of nurse, doctor and dentist and even that non-nurses prescribe and treat. One example is the role and function of the "rig medic" who after brief but specific training is able to carry out quite a wide range of activities in the isolation of a North Sea Oil Rig (albeit with radio access to medical advice). It is worth examining whether in the conventional settings of hospital and surgery, a medical aide could ease the workload of, and therefore make better use of, doctors.

In the United States of America the role of allied health workers has been expanding rapidly during recent years in response to widespread demands for cost effectiveness in the delivery of medical care. Currently, more than 2,500 training programmes for allied health workers are approved by the American Medical Association, and this work-force is expected to increase from approximately 900,000 workers in 1971 to 1.3 million workers by 1980.

Also, physicians themselves are beginning to allow increasing numbers of these workers to perform primary care functions in order to make medical services more widely available. (18) One group of such workers, for example, hospital corpsmen, constitute the largest group of paramedical personnel in the United States Navy. They perform such diverse functions as screening and diagnosing health problems of outpatients, giving emergency treatment to severely ill or injured patients, providing nursing care for hospitalized patients, running laboratory tests and operating radiological equipment, maintaining health records, and supervising other health care personnel. They comprise approximately 80 per cent of the Navy's Medical Department manpower.

Some experience with non-physician health workers in the United States of America has been gained already. (19)

> For example, in out-of-hospital care with stable chronic adult patients an appropriate nursing role is personal support of the patient and medical surveillance of his chronic

disorders and treatment. Care is shared with the doctor when clinical severity increases. Similar definitions for the care of developing children, the sick child and the chronic psychiatric patients have been made.

It is hoped that:

workers will not simply facilitate the intro-duction of technical innovation alone but will rather increase the social dimension of medical care that provides the patient relief, rehabilitation, and optimal maintenance and makes his reception, examination and advice unhurried and his total experience of care and treatment more personal than it now is.

The Soviet Union has had feldshers with a clearly defined role for many years, but most countries with an orthodox health service and large and powerful medical profession have resisted the introduction of physician assistants. Some progress has been made in introducing dental assistants, (20) but there is a less clearly defined nursing service within dentistry, and the supervision and activities of these dental assistants have been strictly laid down.
A comprehensive review of the Physician Assistant (21) covering the literature and an analysis of forty-five programmes in the United States shows some of the changes taking place. There is a move from being a physician's 'assistant' to a physicians's 'associate' and that this involves a sharing in the medical tasks, rather than acceptance of tasks passed on by the doctor. The emphasis on competency based education may have encouraged an examination of physician training. There are however problems of status, legal variables, role irregularity and legitimacy which require to be examined before there is further advance.

THE CHANGING ROLE OF THE NURSE

"... Everybody wants to meet the health manpower shortages by re-designing the role of the nurse ... The role of the nurse is the battleground for job definition within the health delivery system." (22) Not only for reasons of staff shortages but for professional, political and other reasons, both those within the nursing profession and people in many other professions and organizations feel that the time has come for a new look at nursing.

Although it has adapted to changing times, the profession has not changed radically since the days of Florence Nightingale, when the fact that most doctors were men and most nurses were women laid the foundations of the relationship between the two professions.

Although there are now more female doctors and more male nurses and although the two sexes are becoming more equal, the 19th Century male-female relationship still dictates the tone of the 20th Century doctor-nurse relationship. Differences in social class, standards of education and training and expectations have in the past contributed to the maintenance of the differences in professional status. In opposition to these traditional influences, there has been the gradual emergence of an academic approach to nursing an examination of the moral aspects of practice and arguments over professional ideology.

Mayers (23) indicates the dilemma:

Concepts of good nursing practice themselves are being subjected to thorough scrutiny. Consumer expectations for care are changing. The affluent are expecting more sophisticated methods of care. The poor are becoming vocal about their medical and health care needs. They want health professionals to show more concern for and understanding of the problem of poverty and ethnic differences. They want to be treated with dignity and respect. The great middle class is feeling the pressures of economic decline and is demanding a dollar's worth of service for each health care dollar that is spent in the face of spiralling health care costs. Nursing, the largest of the health care professions, must face its responsibilities in all of these and in many more problems.

In addition, the nursing profession itself is beset by internal problems. Changing consumer needs, rapidly advancing medical technology, new communication systems, and new paramedical disciplines are causing many traditional roles and values to crumble, resulting in a sense of confusion and disagreement about who the nurse is and what she does. (There is a swing toward specialization in areas where highly developed technical skill is required, such as in intensive care, renal dialysis and coronary monitoring. There is a growing demand for clinical specialists in psychiatric nursing, medical-surgical nursing and other clinical specialities. On the other hand, the concept of the nurse as a generalist is being widely discussed. Nursing's responsibility for assuming some traditional physican's functions, such as primary diagnostic screening, routine medical evaluat- ions, and counselling is being developed and implemented). Many nurses feel challenged and stimulated by the potentials for change. Others feel concern for a loss of the long and dearly held values and traditions of nursing practice ... in the changing climate of health care, nursing is steadily developing a sense of its multi-dimensional role in delivering health care ... nursing shares roles and responsibil- ities with many other disciplines, in addition, nursing has a unique role, one it shares with no other health care discipline. It is the role of assisting a patient with his ongoing, minute- by-minute, day-by-day personal care mainten- ance, comfort, and safety that is unique to nursing ... very broadly, yet basically stated, nursing is a rational and systematic process which deliberately influences the health- illness ecology so as to maximize the possibility of maintaining personal health, safety, comfort and higher levels of wellness for individuals and groups.

The need for the nurse to function as a change agent or as a patient advocate is clearly put by Kosnik (24)

Nursing can expand roles, change names, and develop new settings in which to work. Yet nursing will be of no value unless we also become politically active in changing our deplorable health and welfare systems, constantly demonstrating humane, patient- centred care regardless of traditional and bureaucratic obstacles. Nursing cannot afford not to allow nurses to become patient advocates.

Common to all new notions of nursing realities referred to earlier is a concern with community nursing. In this context, the following terms are frequently used - "family nurse practitioner", "community nursing", "the extended role of the nurse", "the expanded role of the nurse" and so on. (25)

There seems to be an implication of continuity of care in the term nurse practitioner. Some see this as being a generalist role while others would desire a specialist role, as in mental health with perhaps an emphasis on episodic care. (26-28) Community nursing encompasses all these groups but is not limited to any one. Moreover, distributive care is comprehensive in that it seeks to treat the whole person and to provide the entire range of nursing services to individuals, families and all special groups in the context of the larger community. Central to the notion of the nurse practitioner is the provision of a service beyond the meeting of individual patient needs and toward a diagnosis and treatment of community health needs. This might include provision of health education, well-baby clinics, day care or improved support facilities of the elderly, psychiatric therapist, care of self-poisoning and the whole range of curative and preventive care in the occupational setting. This diagnosis of community health needs involves the nurse practitioner in health planning and evaluation at all levels from planning with a given family to planning for a district.

In a recent article (29) Marion Ferguson discusses the nurse practitioner now found in the United States, who is: "occupying a position somewhere in between the model of the 'traditional physician' and that of the 'traditional nurse'. This new role might be one of the needs of present day society." In the United States, the nurse practitioner:

> takes medical histories, completes physical examinations on patients and interprets various laboratory tests and procedures and becomes highly skilled in preventive medicine. In some places the nurse practitioner also provides extensive care to those who are ill or injured. A difference is made between an <u>associate</u> of the physician and an assistant to the physician ... an associate capable of a high degree of decision-making and practising with consider-able independence.

Marion Ferguson sees the introduction of the practitioner not only as a more efficient use of personnel but also as an opportunity to inject into

the health care system a new way of looking at
health, illness and treatment.

The nurse practitioner by seeing herself as the
patient's advocate could act in many ways as the
pointer for future emphasis in health care
delivery. Her concern for the total needs of her
patient should direct her research interests
into the nature of what consitutes clincial
care. By virtue of her broad based educational
background the nurse practitioner should be
able to recognize sociological, psychological
and biological phenomena as they influence
prognostic development. The backup services she
may need to carry out her patient-centred
nursing care plan may call for a different
method of administrative organization as a
rigid bureaucractic model appears to militate
against personalized patient care.

If patient participation is going to
necessitate a new way of thinking among the
professionals, and an input of personnel with more
diverse training, an extension of the role of the
nurse would seem an appropriate development. The
nursing profession itself, however, will have to
clarify its own position with regard to nursing
duties and functions if there is to be an opportunity
for innovation. Clarification is required as to the
legal implications of these new responsibilities and
then to the training that is most appropriate. (30)

THE VOLUNTEER — NEGLECTED AND MISUNDERSTOOD

We include volunteers in the discussion of task
substitution within the professional section rather
than in that concerning lay participation and self-
help because volunteers, as they are ordinarily
understood, are not also the patients concerned.

The essential element to patient participation
is that patients seek to assume power and responsibility over their own health, thus altering the
traditional helper-helped roles. The volunteer, on
the other hand, gives his or her services to the
professionals, for them to deploy as they see fit,
they are, then, firmly on the 'helper' side of the
barrier.

There has been a long tradition, particularly in
Britain, of encouraging the participation of
volunteers and voluntary groups in health, welfare,

social problems, education, nursing etc. Indeed some of the now recognized and established services either started as voluntary organizations or still have a voluntary component – the ambulance service and blood transfusion service provide two examples.

There has been a tendency in more recent years, particularly with the widespread and comprehensive services available under the welfare state, to regard such voluntary provisions as irrelevant or unnecessary and to denigrate those who provide such services as do-gooders, or middle class ladies with nothing better to do. It became fashionable to sneer at the patronising nature of such work and to regard charities with distrust. Such an approach does not recognize the very real contribution that can be made to health problems, nor does it recognize the sense of fulfillment that it may provide to those who are the volunteers.

Two important factors have led to a review of this position – the recognition that services cannot provide all the range of help and support that is required (this includes both the financial constraints and the inappropriateness of meeting such needs as friendship) and the growing population of people with time and interest who are not in employment.

Of course such work needs considerable skill and probably some training. It does seem however that, throughout the Western world, the days of full employment are gone forever. Increased mechanisation is resulting in a gradual decrease of the working week. People will retire younger and live longer. All this leaves a substantial pool of latent energy, which could be usefully employed as volunteers. It is important to recognize the benefits for the helper as well as the helped and to build on this need to be needed.

It should be added that there are two politico-social 'scenarios' within which this use of the unemployed for voluntary work can occur. Such a process could occur in an avowedly high-technology, low labour-intensive economy where structural unemployment is planned and accepted and which accords the unemployed proper civic status and a concomitant income: this context could see the constructive and long-term marrying of citizens' needs for a defined role in their society and society's need for the performance of various service tasks.

The use of the unemployed in voluntary work can, however, occur in a society where politicians –

officially, at least - see unemployment as temporary
and aberrant. This confers a 'misfit' label upon
those visited by the misfortune of unemployment and
so associates voluntary work by the unemployed with
the general economic depression, welfare cutbacks,
low income and poor status and, consequently, a
perception that the unemployed are being used as
cheap labour by a struggling society. Indeed, some
commentators have believed this latter situation to
be the rationale behind 'community care' releasing
the old and handicapped from paid care into the
unpaid care of the unemployed.

As we have seen, there is room for reallocation
of tasks within the 'helper' camp and this includes
volunteers. If carefully employed, volunteers can
increase the sphere within which to spread the
workload and be used on projects which would not
otherwise be initiated.

Many of the long established voluntary organizations and charities, such as Women's Royal Voluntary
Service and Age Concern still meet a vital need.
Some have altered their function or their titles with
changing social situations. These organizations are
likely to face an increasing demand for their
services as current economic constraints reduce the
availablity of statutory service provision. Other
groups have become redundant after the state has
taken over what they initiated, while others have
continued to act as pressure groups. Some
organizations, particularly those concerned with
long stay hospital patients or specific categories of
disability have continued to provide, quietly and
unobtrusively, friendship, advice and sometimes
small financial or fringe benefits.

New groups have also developed and these usually
seek to provide friendship and support to clearly
defined health problems. In the United States of
America (31) there are examples of volunteers running
educational and screening programmes, alongside
professionals. Two such schemes are at the Lennox
Hill Hospital, New York City and at the Anaheim
(California) Memorial Hospital. At the Memorial
Sloan-Kettering Cancer Centre, New York City,
volunteers now run a patient advocacy programme,
visiting readmitted cancer patients, with the
intention of giving some measure of security and
alleviation of fears and also helping to readjust to
the hospital and treatment. Also in the United States
there has been an emphasis on using older, but
relatively fit people in a number of different ways.
(32) The transition from hospital to community is a

clearly recognized time of uncertainty and anxiety and the possible contribution of volunteers at this critical point has been noted. (33)

One or two studies (34-35) have compared the help given by volunteers with no training with some of the more professionally trained personnel in certain aspects of rehabilitation and little difference has been found. This does not underestimate the value of the various trained therapists – speech, occupational or physician – but shows that regular support and encouragement may be the most important factor at certain stages of the recovery process.

An interesting example where there is obviously mutual help is that of the bereaved and lonely person who after the death of a spouse in hospital continues to visit another lonely hospital patient with chronic or terminal illness. (36) Sometimes the support given by a voluntary group is directed to the support of relatives of patients rather than the patients themselves, e.g. in dementia. (37) There is an opportunity for experimentation and evaluation of these and other similar approaches.

THE PHARMACIST

The significance of medication (both over-the-counter products and prescribed drugs) was indicated in an earlier chapter. There is therefore a clear need for any individual, particularly those on some form of continuing or repeated medication to have information about the appropriate indications, the effects, the duration of treatment, the side effects and the possible interactions of both prescribed and over-the-counter medicine. The present and future contribution of the pharmacist is currently a matter of debate. The relationship between pharmacist and physician is one of the longest standing links in health care, (38) but one that is still uncertain, although it looks as if a new partnership with an emphasis on the educational role of the pharmacist may develop.

For those who prescribe there is a need to ensure that as far as possible, medication is safe, appropriate and necessary, that it is correctly dispensed, that it is being properly taken by the patient and that every effort is made to reduce risks and to detect as soon as possible any side effects. (39) Traditionally, the pharmacist has had a particular responsibility for the proper dispensing of such medications. Another long established function, although less official has been the giving of advice to those who come to a chemists. While this generally consists of requests for a suitable medication for symptoms, the range of problems brought can be very wide, especially in a community where the pharmacist is well known and respected. Although this is easily noted from casual eavesdropping in any chemists shop, the range of problems, the type of advice given and the remedies recommended have been carefully documented. (40,41)

The present debate centres around two main issues. The first concerns the role of the pharmacist in patient education for those on prescribed drugs. Should the pharmacist have a more direct role, building on the traditional dispensing function in providing detailed information on the drug, its use, side effects, etc., and then continuing to have a survelliance or monitoring function - providing continuing contact? The second area of debate, is whether or not the pharmacist should provide a first line of professional care and advice, formalising and expanding the long established unofficial role.

While some contend that both these functions should clearly be the responsibility of the general practitioner, there is considerable support for the idea of these being undertaken by the pharmacist. Others have suggested that a combined approach, using the various staff involved in primary care, the pharmacist and also the hospital staff, is also appropriate.

Both in Britain and in the United States, (42-43) there is pressure from pharmacists for an expanded role - either in clinical pharmacy or community pharmacy. Two reports in Britain have defined the desired future functions. (44-45) Among the more radical proposals are that patients should be required to register with a particular pharmacy for dispensing prescriptions, that pharmacists should keep patient medication records, and that a limited counter prescribing service might be introduced by pharmacists with a patient registration scheme.

The pharmacist of the future will, it is suggested, advise both doctors and patients about prescribed medicines, monitor adverse drug reactions, consult with doctors about prescribing and dispensing procedures, advise members of the public about over-the-counter medicines, and expand his or her function in primary care. Pharmacists may also contribute to health education, take part in diagnostic screening procedures and provide domiciliary pharmaceutical services to housebound patients and nursing homes. The pharmacist is easily available and approachable. He or she can advise patients whether to take over-the-counter medicines or to see the doctor. Since most chemists sell a variety of goods besides drugs, patients will often call at the shop and can be observed for effects of medication.

As a result of a survey, Pilkington (46) concludes that there is quite a strong demand by the public for the general practice pharmacists to undertake an official and expanded role in the advisory field of health education and health maintenance. Harris (47) from his study of pharmacists found that they were equally eager to become involved in health education. Involvement in family planning, smoking cessation, child health and advice on immunization have been specifically proposed. Even when their advice is not sought, they could intervene and not allow the distraught teenager to buy three bottles of asprin or the down-and-out to buy 'meths', but could refer them to more effective methods of help.

The report by the Pharmaceutical Society indicated that pharmacists are interested in this extension of their work. Perhaps it could be recognized formally that the pharmacist not only dispenses but also treats and advises and his training and income could be adjusted accordingly; this might stem the present rapid loss of corner chemist shops.

There is of course the possible complication that the pharmacist gains financially from some treatments and not from others and advice may be biased accordingly. The same is true, however, of other professionals and although abuse cannot be ruled out, it may be that professional ethics and the fact that the pharmacist in the corner shop is very much a local figure with relationships and responsibilities in that community, will control any conflicts of interest.

More than ten years ago Whitfield (40) concluded from a study that the advice given by pharmacists to the public was of a good standard and that they relieved general practitioners of a great deal of work. However, there is still considerable opposition by the medical profession (48) to this expanded role and function: "Despite strong reservations by the B.M.A., plans are moving ahead for a clinical trial in which pharmacists will actually treat patients for minor illnesses."

This unfavourable response is unlikely to lead to a better liaison between doctor and pharmacist or to a reduction in the discontent expressed by many pharmacists at present. In particular it will not lead to improved care for patients. A cautious, but more balanced approach is contained in the British Medical Journal editorial: (43)

> Hospital pharmacists are not faced with the same commercial dilemma as their colleagues in general practice. Even so, any move to expand the role of either hospital or community pharmacists will inevitably encounter resistance as it encroaches on the traditional territories of doctors and nurses. Hospital pharmacy is, however, making progress with the development of ward pharmacy and drug information centres - a change whose impetus came from the Noel Hall Report in 1970, which asserted that 'the hospital pharmacist today has a continuing and heavy responsibility for ensuring with his medical and nursing colleagues that drugs are used safely, effectively and economically'.
>
> Without doubt deficiencies exist in the application of knowledge about drugs to the everyday treatment of patients, in the education of doctors about drugs, and in the information given to patients, who are often left in total ignorance about their disorders and their treatment. Hence there is a good case for hoping that doctors should look forward to any contribution that future pharmacists might make to the safe use of medicines. But future pharmacists must also recognize the clinical knowledge and skills of the doctor and his ultimate responsibility for the care of his patients and must understand that drugs are part of a patient's treatment. Drug prescribing cannot be considered in isolation: diagnosis and treatment are interdependent.
>
> The new generalist and specialist roles for the pharmacist will have to evolve slowly, for both pharmacists and doctors will need to recognize that there are substantial differences between present knowledge and skills and those required for these expanded functions. The speed and ease of the evolutionary process will depend on how much doctors encourage pharmacists to take on their new

responsibilities in patient care and how much each is willing to contribute to the other's education and training. Many of the problems faced by pharmacists have been created by their educational isolation from health care – compounded by their not speaking the language of doctors or sharing their medical knowledge. This communication gap can be closed if pharmacists learn about diseases and their treatment and are given the opportunity to learn and practice alongside doctors and nurses. But pharmacy education is not yet geared to meet such demands. Pharmacists of the future will need their undergraduate courses revised and lengthened, and they will want graduate training programmes and provisions for continuing education and career structures for pharmacists in clinical services.

Like medicine and nursing, pharmacy is in transition. Both pharmacists and doctors need to remember that whatever problems there are in dispensing and prescribing in the NHS have not been created by any one group and are not going to be solved by any one group. Without the help of doctors the expanded role of pharmacists will not develop nor will it develop if doctors feel threatened rather than recognizing that future pharmacists could complement their services to their patients. In the future, pharmacists, doctors, and nurses should be less concerned with the protection of professional boundaries and territories and more concerned with patient care.

A NEW ROLE

So far in this chapter we have indicated some developments that may include changing roles for existing personnel roles, but a further few examples may illustrate the more innovative changes that are taking place. These include completely new roles, services offered in a different way, increased responsibility in a professional group, taking over new functions or retreiving functions that it had previously.

Counselling provides an example of a new role. Some of the skills and activities have been carried out in the past by older established professional groups and indeed are still practised by these groups today – social workers, psychiatrists and psychologists. Counselling services which are specially set up may either be in association with an established service or be completely separated. The Isis Centre (49) is an example of one, closely linked with existing psychiatric services, but referral may be from general practitioners or other agencies or clients may refer themselves. Similar types of services are related to the problems of addiction.

Most discussion has centred around the problems of young people - is there need for an independent confidential consulting service for problems relating to school, family, leisure, sex or work? This has been reviewed by Orchard, (50) who after careful consideration felt that existing professional health and education services did not and probably could not provide an acceptable service of help and support.

Voluntary Service Overseas is the provision of skills, but in a different way from usual. In the 19th and early part of the 20th Century there was a clear recognition of the health needs of developing countries by the various religious organizations. This resulted in a rapid expansion in medical missionary work - combining medical care with the proclamation of the religious, usually Christian, faith. In many countries this has continued to provide not only treatment, but also the education and training of health workers. More recently there has been a tendency for young people at the beginning of their professional careers to offer their services overseas. In addition to doctors and nurses, many other skills are required to help overcome the problems of the developing countries - nutritionists, therapists of various kinds, auxiliaries, technicians, etc. New policies for this type of contribution are now being worked out. (51)

Recent developments in clinical psychology illustrate an increase in professional independence for psychologists. They are now undertaking independent patient care whereas previously, clinical psychologists were seeing only those patients referred by the doctor. Another change taking place is the move from centralised hospital bases to a community orientation: pilot studies are examining the contribution of a clinical psychologist as part of the primary care team. (52) Similarly expanded and more independent functions are now found amongst dietitians.

THE ENVIRONMENT

In 1976 the World Health Organization reported (53) that 62% of the population of developing countries did not have reasonable access to a safe water supply and 68% had inadequate facilities for the sanitary disposal of human excretion. This 62% represents 1,250 million people. To those in the developed countries who benefit from the pioneer work of John Snow and the Sanitary Movement of the 19th Century, and takes for granted such facilities, these figures illustrate the discrepancy between the developed and developing countries.

At Habitat, the United Nations Conference on Human Settlements, 1976(54) it was recommended that programmes should be adopted to provide water for all urban and rural areas by 1980 if at all possible. It was also recommended that programmes for the sanitary disposal of excreta and waste water in urban and rural areas should be adopted and accelerated. The following year at the United Nations Water Conference (55) these recommendations were reiterated and it was advocated that the decade 1980-1990 should be designated as "The International Drinking Water Supply and Sanitation Decade" and that it should be devoted to implementing the national plans for drinking water supply and sanitation.

Ballance (56) points out:

> the provision of physical facilities is, by itself, not enough. Health education in the sanitary handling of water and wastes, a potentially potent tool, has yet to be widely used for the successful control of disease.

He notes that while a great deal can be done by applying existing technological knowledge, there is a real need for study of the socio-cultural dimensions of technological interventions for water supply and sanitation. This would yield information on how to encourage a greater involvement of individuals in the planning and construction of systems and thus generate an improved understanding of what they, their families and their community have to gain through improved sanitation. Finally, he considers that current technical information should be more widely available to engineers, sanitarians, rural development workers and primary health workers, preferably in their own languages.

In the developed countries until recently the environmental aspects of health have been taken for granted - something which had been achieved and was no longer of interest or concern. Public health was regarded as old fashioned, low status and produced jokes about rats and drains. This was epitomised in the change from public Health to Community Medicine - with the conventional aspects being largely forgotten. Recently there has been a renewal of interest - firstly from concerned groups in the community who have drawn attention to wide aspects of ecology, pollution and conservation. Belatedly professional groups and those with administrative responsibility are slowly following this lead. (57)

The link between environment, both physical and social and health, has been recognized since the early days of civilization. Hippocrates in his "Air, Water and Places" referred to this important relationship. The effects of city life, housing conditions, overcrowding, opportunities for leisure and recreation and atmospheric pollution have all been intensively studied. (58-60) The possible harmful effects of toxic substances on human beings, animals and the environment are now topics of concern in the media and the subject of discussion in most sectors of the community. This applies not only to the workplaces where these potentially hazardous substances are manufactured, but also to other occupational situations where they may be used and to the possible chance exposure of the general public or consumer when at home or at work. (61-62) In these latter settings there is frequently little awareness or understanding of the risk or the need for special precautions. The place-names of major industrial disasters Minnimata, Flixborough and Seveso are now well known and act as a warning.

Some products which were designed to improve health or to control disease have themselves been found to be harmful to health. Pesticides not only can have a harmful effect on the human beings who use them (if they are not handled with great care) but they can contaminate foodstuffs causing poisonings and they can have widespread harmful effects on birds and animals in the environment. (63-64)

In considering the working environment it is necessary to take account not only of the materials in use but also the manner of their use. A product may not be used in the way anticipated by the manufacturer. There is now a responsibility on the manufacturer, under the Health and Safety at Work Act (65) to ensure that the article or substance is safe and without risk to health when properly used and to make available necessary information to encourage proper use. New knowledge may require a reappraisal of existing practice. The possible carcinogenic and teratogenic effects of existing components and newly introduced substances is one of the most urgent areas of concern. The serious effects of vinyl chloride monomer exemplify the need for continuing vigilance. New technological problems such as those developed for the North Sea Oil industry bring new problems - both physical and social for those who work in such abnormal environments. (66)

Early detection of hazards, clear assessment of the risks involved and a high index of suspicion provides the best approach to the control of environmental health problems. The need to balance the risks (and often there is only a suspicion of risk) with the significant contribution such products and industries make to society presents a clear challenge to those involved in social policy. (67-69)

Not only in the field of the physical environment is there a concern, but interest in improving the overall quality of life is widespread. Herzberg (70) sums up the dilemma: for the first time in history we have the opportunity to satisfy man's inherent wants. Yet what value is there to people if industry manufactures commodities to supply material comfort at the expense of development and happiness. The social and intellectual aspects of work also have implications for health. While the fortunate few can speak of free choice of employment, opportunity and satisfaction, many workers find, as Tredgold (71) points out, that their work is soul destroying, frustrating or boring; when there is no challenge, no purpose, no sense of achievement, it may be necessary to find one's satisfaction elsewhere. In contrast to those who suffer as a result of lack of stimulus in the work situation there are those who suffer from excessive demands and overwork and those who find work too demanding or too challenging. (72)

The dynamic nature of the relationship between people and their environment has been clearly stated by Dubos. (73) Surprisingly little attention has been paid to the enormous implications for health of industrialisation and urbanisation nor has the relationship between health and rapid social change been examined with sufficient care. The place and purpose of work in contemporary society and the many different environmental influences on health require clarification.

Self-help groups (74) have developed in industry, involving trade unions, Workers' Educational Associations and various academics.

Their aim is to increase information, improve communication, provide a reference library and carry out industrial surveys. Officially appointed under the Health and Safety at Work Act, Safety Representatives (75) may in future make a significant contribution to improving health and safety. It is to be hoped that these moves will lead to an increased awareness of this aspect of the working environment in the unions. In addition to those in management with responsibility for health and safety, doctors, nurses, first aiders and occupational hygienists play a significant role. The key role is that of the nurse with a training in occupational health, who takes responsibility for diagnosis and treatment; undertakes evaluation of the working environment; acts as a health educator, provides a counselling function and administers a 24 hour emergency cover service. This is an obvious example of an expanded and changing role. (76) It is however unlikely that much will be achieved until everyone in industry is concerned and trained to be their own on-the-job inspector and is given an opportunity to participate in decision making. (77-78) The Trades Union Congress (79) has recently sought to stimulate discussion through proposals for more comprehensive services for a greater proportion of the working population.

Increasingly the need to assess the effects of any planning exercise on health and environment is being recognized. This includes the immediate and the long-term effects of nuclear power, the production of natural resources and environmental conservation, the re-use of water and wastes, and in the developing countries the increase in malaria and schistosomiasis from irrigation schemes.(80) Clearly in these and many other issues described in this chapter there is a requirement for health professionals to work in partnership with other professionals and non-professionals.

> Physicians must learn to work with engineers, architects and general biologists, as well as with city planners, lawyers and politicians responsible for the management of our social life. Only through such collaboration can they help society ward off, insofar as possible, dangers to physical and mental health inherent in all technological and social changes, especially when these occur as rapidly as they do now. From urban renewal to safety measures in industry, from environmental pollution, to the trial of new drugs and therapeutic

procedures, the sociomedical problems are countless and require technical, legal and ethical consideration. (81)

THE TEAM APPROACH TO HEALTH - IS THIS THE ANSWER?

It is fashionable at present to talk of the multi-disciplinary team and to make the assumption that this will be the answer to professional problems and the community's needs. Some multidisciplinary teams (82) are now involved in deciding on admission and discharge policies and principles governing medication and treatment - areas previously the sole prerogative of the consultant in charge. Teams may be able to overrule the doctor with respect to decisions on the care of patients. Often, however the competitive elements can over-rule the co-operative ideal. Some understanding of what the word "profession" stands for may lead to a better idea of the conflicts that may be inherent in any such team and that sometimes more attention is paid to maintaining professional integrity than the meeting of public need or demand.

George Bernard Shaw's statement (83) that "every profession is a conspiracy against the laity" is well known, but why does a profession such as medicine which is ostensibly scientific, altruistic and pre-occupied with the relief of suffering and the saving of life, still call forth such remarks? A profession is distinguished by its body of specialized knowledge, is monopoly, autonomy and its self regulation. As Freidson (84) points out, the medical profession, which is the prototype profession is noted for its pre-eminence in prestige and expert authority and this is enhanced by its area of concern - of life and death - of intimate personal and psychological areas and its spiritual and emotional overtones. Inevitably this long established profession finds it difficult to cope with changing social demands, emergent new professionals and patients and a public who seek new roles. And yet it is well-known how rapidly new medical techniques are superceded and discarded: it is evident that the medical profession welcomes progress, scientific advances, change. In what sense can it be said that doctors are resistant to change?

The anthropologist, Radcliffe-Brown (85) differentiates two kinds of social change. The first - 're-adjustment' - is the sort which occurs in the normal course of events. At a marriage, for instance, a regrouping of people takes place, a new family develops and so, in some sense there has been change. But it could be said that the pattern of marriage and family grouping has thereby been conserved and reinforced, not at all changed. The second sort of change - 'change of type' - is when the structural form of society alters. Professionals in the medical sphere are committed to changes within the system - readjustments but without any alteration in the general roles, status and rules. Many individuals and groups in the community (and indeed some of the newer professional groups) however, would seek a much more dramatic 'change of type' - with a shift in the balance of power and a readjustment of the equilibrium of the social structure. Thus it can be seen that the medical profession does indeed espouse change in one sense - in the form of new drugs etc. but is resistent to changes which threaten its pre-eminence in the health care system.

In addition to some of the challenges to change already mentioned there is a direct challenge to the medical profession from alternative therapies such as osteopaths and chiropracters. The relationship between such groups, the state and the medical profession are being examined. (86-88) The influence of such alternatives and their popularity may have resulted in the increased interest within the medical profession in such measures as manipulative medicine. (89)

Whereas it is relatively easy for academics and planners in the west to talk of introducing new categories of primary health care in developing countries, the implications of this along with the increased emphasis on self-care may also have an impact on primary care in the developed countries. (90) Saint-Yves (91) has suggested a new system of primary care in Britian in which suitably trained health staff - most likely nurses - would provide a fully comprehensive, continuous, caring, prevention-oriented system in which the general practitioner woud act as a "specialist" generalist. Further experiments are required to evaluate the acceptability of a system where the general practitioner need not be the patients' first contact with the health service.

The participation of patients in practice groups involved in policy making decisions and patients and relatives being included as full team members in providing individual care are a considerable departure from normal medical practice in Britain. (92-93) The British Medical Assocation is gradually recommending the recognition of self-help groups and their contribution in health care and is suggesting that doctors should be trained in counselling techniques. (94)

It is not surprising that it should be necessary to have a paper entitled "A Patient's Charter" published in the British Medical Journal in 1979. (95) This proposes a few basic rules to ensure that patients and relatives are not treated as if they were less responsible, adult and intelligent than those caring for them. The author concludes the article as follows:

> The practical measures I have suggested will bring comfort to the patient and boost his morale: but they will not be enough unless there are also changes of bias in educational aims and understanding of the power and range of factors that determine patient care. The achievement of these objectives might seem a daunting task, but to do nothing means turning a blind eye to behaviour that falls short of acceptable levels at times, has a damaging effect on professional well-being, and places an added burden on patients. As doctors we are not different from our patients despite our efforts to prove otherwise, so that enlightened self-interest if nothing else should provide a powerful incentive towards improving the quality and consistency of care.

An example from Australia (96) shows the types of initiative that are possible which incorporate research, team approach and community participation. In a Brisbane suburb, following an epidemiological survey which was mainly concerned with the health care of young children and their mothers - a programme directly based on the results of the study was produced. This was the product of the combined efforts of the research team (well known to the community and accepted by them after three years of research) and the participants.

The aim was to achieve the knowledge, skills and values being the following capacities:
1.   Participating actively and knowledgeably in one's own health care;
2.   Being able to make a balanced decision on which services to use and when to use them;
3.   Being able to talk over a health problem with a health adviser;
4.   Being able to take care, appropriately, of minor

emergencies and self-limiting illness without using the services;
5.   Being able to report the history and status of a health problem, either in a surgery or over the telephone;
6.   Being able to select appropriate medications from pharmacies, and appreciate their individual effectiveness;
7.   Being able to recognize health hazards and health risks in the home (and locally) and undertake appropriate measures (as far as is possible) to reduce the level of health risk;
8.   Being able to recognize what is normal (as opposed to average) and what isn't in the areas of child development and growth (physically, socially, emotionally and behaviourally);
9.   Feeling confident in oneself when health problems arise and in dealing with them (understanding too, that "getting sick" occasionally is a normal part of life and need not be accompanied by feelings of failure or guilt);
10.   Being able to help each other through some socially supportive network, especially in the practical problems of underservices suburban living.

The importance of establishing a credible base in this participatory activity was noted. This was aided by the similarity in life cycle stage between members of the research team and the participants, and the similarity in service's use at the local level. The authors refer to the concept of "health field" showing health status as a function of the interaction of human biology, environment, lifestyle and health care organization. Such an ecological approach has implications for change in the societal systems and manifests a more radical approach than selective prevention.

This chapter has highlighted some of the changes and the problems – but the solutions are yet to be worked out. Much will depend on the attitudes of the professionals, their willingness to adapt and to be innovative and to the education offered to their successors. As Dubos points out there is an exciting opportunity. (97)

> The role of medicine is to help man function well, as long as feasible, and if possible, happily in all his endeavours – whether he is toiling for his daily bread, creating urban civilization, writing a poem, or attempting to reach the moon. These examples are not taken at random; they symbolize the worlds of nature,

thought, feeling and technology.

Medicine was, at the beginning of civilization, the mother of sciences, and played a large role in the integration of early cultures. Later, it constituted the bridge over which science and humanism maintained some contact. Today, it has once more the opportunity of becoming a catalytic force in civilization by pointing to the need, and providing the leadership, for the development of a science of man.

The continued growth of technological civilization, indeed its very survival, requires an enlargement of our understanding of man's nature. Man can function well only when his external environment is in tune with the needs he has inherited from his evolutionary, experimental, and social past, and with his aspirations for the future. Because they are concerned with all the various aspects of man's humanness, the biomedical sciences in their highest form are potentially the richest expression of science.

NOTES

1. Mahler H. World Health is Indivisible. Interdisciplinary Science Reviews 1978; 3, No 3: 178-180.
2. Mahler H. Foreword in Elliott K. (Ed.) Auxiliaries in Primary Health Care. An Annotated Bibliography London: Intermediate Technology Publications, 1979.
3. Elliott K. (Ed.) Auxiliaries in Primary Health Care. An Annotated Bibliography London: Intermediate Technology Publications, 1979.
4. Gish O. Doctor Auxiliaries in Tanzania. Lancet 1973; 2: 1251-1252.
5. Chagula WK. & Tarimo E. Meeting Basic Health Needs in Tanzania. In Newell WK. (Ed.) Health by the People Geneva: World Health Organization, 1975, 145-168.
6. Ministry of Health, United Republic of Tanzania. Primary Health Care - Tanzania Experience. International Conference on Primary Health Care.
7. Ministry of Health, Democratic Republic of the Sudan. Primary Health Care Programme -Eastern, Northern, Central and Western Regions of Sudan 1977/78 - 1983/84 Khartoum: Khartoum University Press, 1976.

8.   Ronaghy HA. Kawar Village Health Worker Project. Tropical Paediatrics and Environmental Child Health 1978; Monograph 52.
9.   Essex BJ. Diagnostic Pathways in Clinical Medicine. An Epidemiological Approach to Clinical Problems Edinburgh: Churchill Livingstone, 1977.
10.   United States Department of Health Education and Welfare. Barefoot Doctor's Manual Washington; Public Helath Services, 1974.
11.   World Health Organization. The Primary Health Worker. Working Guide, Guidelines for Training, Guidelines for Adoption Geneva: World Health Organization, 1977.
12.   Abbatt FR. Teaching for Better Learning Genevea: World Health Organization, 1980.
13.   Bennett FJ. Primary Health Care and Developing Countries. Social Science and Medicine 1979; 13A: 505-514.
14.   Smith KA. Health Promotion in the Poorer Countries. Social Science and Medicine 1975; 9: 121-132.
15.   World Health Organization. The Promotion and Development of Traditional Medicine: Report of a Meeting Technical Report Series No. 662. Geneva: World Health Organization, 1978.
16.   Montageau B., Smith HL. and Mawey AC. The "Granny" Midwife - Changing Roles and Functions of a Folk Practitioner. American Journal of Sociology 1961; 66: 497-505.
17.   Maclean U. Ethnic Healing. Medical Education 1979; 13: 241.
18.   Booth RF., Webster EG. and McNally MS. Schooling, Occupational Motivation and Personality as Related to Success in Paramedical Training. Public Health Reports 1976; 91: 533-537.
19.   Stoeckle JD. and Twaddle AC. Non-physician Health Workers: Some Problems and Prospects. Social Science and Medicine 1974; 8: 71-76.
20.   Holt RD. and Murray JJ. An Evaluation of the Role of New Cross Dental Auxiliaries and of Their Clinical Contribution to the Community Dental Services. Parts I & II. British Dental Journal 1980; 149: 227-230 and 259-262.
21.   Schneller ES. The Physicians Assistant Lexington: DC Heath, 1978.
22.   Gorshenson C. Trends in Health Care: An Interview. Maternal and Child Care Health Information 1970; Vol.4 No. 2.
23.   Mayers MG. A Systematic Approach to the Nursing Care Plan New York: Appleton, 1973.
24.   Kosik SH. Patient Advocacy of Fighting the

System. In Spradley BW. (Ed.) <u>Contemporary Community Nursing</u> Boston: Little Brown, 1975.

25. Marks IM., Connolly J. and Hallam RG. Psychiatric Nurse as Therapist. <u>British Medical Journal</u> 1973; 3: 156-160.

26. Marks IM., Connolly J. and Hallam RG. Psychiatric Nurse as Therapist. <u>British Medical Journal</u> 1973; 3: 156-160.

27. Editorial. Policies on Self-Poisoning. <u>British Medical Journal</u> 1979; 2: 1091-1092.

28. Clark J. (i) Diagnosis and Prescribing by Nurses. (ii) When Should Nurses Prescribe? <u>Occupational Health</u> 1978; 30: 12-15 and 60-63.

29. Ferguson MC. Nursing at the Cross-Roads. Which Way to Turn? A Look at the Model of Nurse Practitioner. <u>Journal of Advanced Nursing</u> 1976; 1/3: 237-242.

30. Department of Health and Society Security. <u>The Extending Role of the Clinical Nurse. Legal Implications and Training Requirements</u> HC(77)27. London: D.H.S.S., 1977.

31. Rockwood B. Myriad of Programmes Serve Well. <u>Hospital - Journal of the American Hospital Association</u> 1976; 50/7: 121-124.

32. Bowles E. Older Persons as Providers of Services. Three Federal Programmes. <u>Social Policy</u> 1976; 7/3: 81-88.

33. Gay P. and Pitkeathley J. <u>When I Went Home ... A Study of Patients Discharged from Hospital</u> London: King Edwards Hospital Fund, 1979.

34. Meikle M., Weschler E., Tupper A., Benenson M., Butler J., Mulhall D., and Stern G. Comparative Trial of Volunteer and Professional Treatments of Dysphasia After Stroke. <u>British Medical Journal</u> 1979; 2: 87-89.

35. Lesser R. and Watt M. Untrained Community Help in the Rehabilitation of Stroke Sufferers with Language Disorder. <u>British Medical Journal</u> 1978; 2: 1045-1048.

36. Radford K. and Wright WB. Can Bereaved Relatives and Hospitals Help One Another. <u>World Medicine</u> 1978; 13 No 10: 53.

37. Fuller J., Ward E., Evans A., Massam K. and Gardner A. Dementia - Supportive Groups for Relatives. <u>British Medical Journal</u> 1979; 1: 1684-1685.

38. Smith MC. The Relationship Between Pharmacy and Medicine. In Mapes R. (Ed.) <u>Prescribing Practice and Drug Usage</u> London: Croom Helm, 1980.

39. Herxheimer A. and Lionel NDW. Minimum Information Needed by Prescribers. <u>British Medical</u>

Journal 1978; 2: 1129-1132.

40. Whitfield M. The Pharmacist's Contribution to Medical Care. The Practitioner 1968; 200: 434-438.

41. Crooks J. and Christopher LJ. Use and Misuse of Home Medicines. In Anderson JAD. Self-Medication Lancaster: M.T.P. Press, 1979.

42. Dickinson K., Novick LF., Loewenstein R., Gretin B., and Asnes RS. Expanded Roles for the Community Pharmacist - Which Direction? Public Health Reports 1976; 91: 226-230.

43. Editorial. Expanding Role for Pharmacists. British Medical Journal 1978; 2: 911-912.

44. Interim Report of the Working Party on the Future of General Practice Pharmacy. Pharmaceutical Journal 1978; 221: 11.

45. Evidence from the Pharmaceutical Society of Great Britain to the Royal Commission on the National Health Service. Pharmaceutical Journal 1977; 218: 72.

46. Pilkington EM. The Role of the General Practice Pharmacist in Health Education and Health Maintenance. Health Education Journal 1979; 39: 187-192.

47. Harris J. An Investigation of the Determinants of the Advisory and Information Service and the Potential for Health Education in Retail Pharmacy Health Education Journal 41: 42-46.

48. Commentary: Should Pharmacists Treat Patients? B.M.A. News Review 1978; 4: 776.

49. Agulnik P., Holroy DP. and Mandelbrote B. The Isis Centre: A Counselling Service Within the National Health Service. British Medical Journal 1976; 2: 355-357.

50. Orchard TJ. The Counselling Needs, Health and Personal Problems of Adolescents M.Med.Sci. Thesis, University of Nottingham, 1978.

51. Voluntary Service Overseas. Health Care in the Third World, A New Policy for V.S.O.

52. Clark DF. The Clinical Psychologist in Primary Care. Social Science and Medicine 1979; 13A: 707-713.

53. World Health Organization. World Health Statistics Report 29 No 10 543-632. Geneva: World Health Organization, 1970.

54. United Nations. Report of Habitat: United Nations Conference on Human Settlements Vancouver 31 May - 11 June 1976. (Document A/Conf 70/15) New York, 1976.

55. United Nations. Report of the United Nations Water Conference Mar Del Plata, 14-25 March 1977. (Document E/Conf 70/29) New York,

1977.
56. Ballance RC. Water Supply, Sanitation and Technology. Interdisciplinary Science Reviews 1978; 3 No 3: 190-195.
57. Unit for the Study of Health Policy. Rethinking Community Medicine. London: U.S.H.P,. 1979.
58. World Health Organization. Health Hazards of the Human Environment Geneva: World Health Organization, 1972.
59. Gray JAM. Housing, Health and Illness. British Medical Journal 1978; 2: 100-101.
60. Downham MAPS., MacGibbon R., Preston GM. and Tyrrell SM. Medical Care in the Inner Cities. British Medical Journal 1978; 2: 545-548.
61. Vouk VB. and Parizek J. Chemicals and Health. Interdisciplinary Science Reviews 1978; 3 No 3: 207-213.
62. Ashby E. Legislation Outside the Factory: The British Philosophy of Pollution Control. In CIBA Foundation Symposium 32 - New Series. Health and Industrial Growth Amsterdam: Elsevier, 1975.
63. Carson R. The Silent Spring New York: Fawcett, 1978.
64. Gratz NG. and Hamon J. Ecology and Vector Control. Interdisciplinary Science Reviews 1978; 3 No 3: 214-219.
65. The Health and Safety at Work Act London: H.M.S.O., 1974.
66. McEwen J. Health and Work. In Sutherland I. (Ed.) Health Education. Perspectives and Choices London: Allen and Unwin, 1979.
67. Society of Occupational Medicine. Proceedings of the Symposium on the Early Detection of Occupational Hazards London: Society of Occupational Medicine, 1971.
68. Society of Occupational Medicine. Proceedings of the Symposium on the Assessment of Exposure and Risk London: Society of Occupational Medicine, 1973.
69. Lee WR. The Assessment of Risks to Health at Work. In Carter C. and Peel J. (Eds.) Equalities and Inequalities in Health London: Academic Press, 1976.
70. Herzberg F. Work and Nature of Man London: Staples Press, 1968.
71. Tredgold RF. Satisfaction at Work or Outside it? Lancet 1971; 2: 420-423.
72. Rhoads JM. Overwork. Journal of the American Medical Association 1977; 237: 2615-2618.
73. Dubos R. Man Adapting New Haven: Yale

University Press, 1965, p.xviii.

74. Feedback. At the Grass Roots of Preventive Medicine. New Scientist 1977; 28 April.

75. Health and Safety Commission. Safety Representatives and Safety Committees London: H.M.S.O., 1977.

76. McDonald JC. Four Pillars of Occupational Health. British Medical Journal 1981; 282: 83-88.

77. Gregory D. and McCarty J. The Shop Stewards' Guide to Workplace Health and Safety Nottingham: Spokesman Books, 1975.

78. Wegman DH., Boden L. and Levenstine C. Health Hazard Surveillance by Industrial Workers. American Journal of Public Health 1975; 45: 26-30.

79. Trades Union Congress. Workplace Health and Safety Services. T.U.C. Proposals for an Integrated Approach London: T.U.C., 1980.

80. World Health Organization. Environmental Health Impact Assessment Report on W.H.O. Seminar. Euro Reports and Studies 7. Copenhagen: World Health Organization, 1979.

81. Dubos R. Man, Medicines and Environemnt London: Pall Mall Press, 1968, p.91.

82. Appleyard J. and Maden JG. Multidisciplinary Teams. British Medical Journal 1979; 2: 1305-1307.

83. Williams P. and Clare A. Social Workers in Primary Health Care: The General Practitioner's Viewpoint. Journal of the Royal College of General Practitioners 1979; 29: 554-558.

84. Freidson E. Profession of Medicine. A Study of the Sociology of Applied Knowledge New York: Dodd Mead, 1972.

85. Radcliffe-Brown AR. Method in Social Anthropology Midway reprint series. Chicago: University of Chicago Press, 1959.

86. Culliton BJ. and Waterfall WK. Chiropractors and the A.H.A. British Medical Journal 1979 1: 467-468.

87. Hocken AG. Chiropractic in From the Cold? British Medical Journal 1980; 281: 97-98.

88. Parliament. Chiropratic and the N.H.S. British Medical Journal 1980; 281: 57.

89. Ebbetts J. The Present Position of Manipulative Medicine. The Practitioner 1979; 222: 798-801.

90. Backett EM. and England R. How Barefoot? Next Steps for the Medical Auxiliary. Lancet 1975; 2: 1137-1138.

91. Saint Yves IFM. Need General Practitioners be Patient's First Contact with Health Service.

Lancet 1980; 2: 578-580.
    92. Goldmeer D., Hollander D. and Sheeham MJ. Relatives and Friends Group in a Psychiatric Ward. British Medical Journal 1979; 1: 932-934.
    93. GMS. Committee. Patient Participation Groups. British Medical Journal 1979; 2: 1160-1161.
    94. Counselling. (a) Self-help Group Plays an Important Role in Tackling Depressive Illness. (b) Training Doctors in New Counselling Techniques. B.M.Λ. News Review 1979; 5: 35.
    95. Zeitlyn BB. A Patient's Charter. British Medical Journal 1979; 2: 1160-1161.
    96. Brownlea A., Taylor C., Lanbeck M. Wishart R. Nalder C. and Behan S. Participatory Health Care: An Experimental Self-helping Project in a Less Advantaged Community. Social Science and Medicine 1980; 14D: 139-146.
    97. Dubos R. Man, Medicine and Environment London: Pall Mall Press, 1968, p.119.

Chapter Thirteen

THE WAY AHEAD

This review has attempted to describe how the notion of participation is affecting health care today. It does not claim to be a comprehensive catalogue but rather a pointer to the many directions in which the idea of participation is taking the health services.

It is intended, however, that this book will provide a basis for further detailed analyses and encourage others to undertake the evaluative research that is so badly lacking. It might also provide the stimulus for people to set up innovative programmes.

Clearly there is a need for:

-   further documentation of existing activities – possibly examining components of this large topic area in greater detail;
-   development of a sound theoretical base;
-   evaluative studies of ongoing activities;
-   setting up well-planned controlled studies to test some of the ideas and to determine the benefits and the hazards of different aspects of participation;
-   determination of health needs and assessment of the tasks required to meet these needs;
-   review of the roles of different health personnel;
-   development, testing and evaluation of educational materials and methods;
-   creation of new models for a more participatory health service.

If participation is to lead to improved health and quality of life, then in the authors' opinion, the following areas present exciting challenges.

SOCIAL INEQUALITIES

Although it is recognized that inequalities in health
(1) are due primarily to economic, social, cultural,
occupational and environmental factors, and that
priority for action must be devoted to these root
causes, it is wrong to go to the extreme of denying
that health services can contribute to health. Morris
(2) refutes such attacks on the health services and
calls for a new partnership between the individual
and society to seek to improve health care.

An over-emphasis on the importance of self-care
may lead to the individual being 'blamed' for his or
her own ill health. (3) The growth of self-help, lay
treatment and community support groups can be seen as
a cheap panacea which allows government and
authorities to shirk their responsibilities and so
should be viewed with caution. And yet to challenge
the social inequalities underlying health problems
is effectively to challenge the government and
authorities and so must logically be the
responsibility of the lay individual and the
community group. Governments and health authorities
are unlikely to challenge themselves.

Clearly there is much that can be done by health
authorities in prevention, treatment and care
('care' so often being neglected in favour of the
more dramatic 'cure' – the challenge of improving
quality of life in terminal care must surely be an
oustanding example). With inner city problems and
other examples of inequality, a radical reallocation
of resources is called for, (4) maximum resources
being given to those with the greatest need.

PROFESSIONAL VERSUS SELF-CARE

"Doctor bashing" has been an acceptable literary
activity for several years. Mahler (5) in his well
known paper in 1975 emphasized the need for
"demystification" and others rightly continue to
point to the deficiency in health care systems and in
professional practice. (6) However, the challenge
now is to attempt to integrate professional and self-
care in the most fruitful way. Backett (7) in a
discussion paper on two articles on self-help (8,9)
succinctly summarises the position: "The increasing
public awareness of the proper limits of professional
health care must be equalled by an awareness of the
terrible effects of no scientifically based health
care at all." Perhaps new terminology will be

helpful. If Levin (8) sees the lay person as the
"primary care practitioner" then Backett's (7) view
of the doctor as a true "consultant" to the patient
is appropriate.

Just as the links between public and
professionals need to be clarified, Godber (10) draws
attention to the importance of a suitable statutory
base on which prevention and health promotion can
build, and that if responsibility is to be shared, it
must be acknowledged that the professionals should
not get all the blame for failures. For too long we
have perpetuated the divisions between those
professionals who, after years of special training,
provide the formal health services and those who
despite their years of experience and their provision
of self-care are regarded as the lay public. "People
are not just consumers of health care, they provide
it themselves". (11)

PRIMARY CARE, PREVENTION AND HEALTH EDUCATION

With the major advances in prevention of acute
disease, the separation in practice between
prevention and care seems increasingly incongruous,
(12) and the integration of these components into
'anticipatory care' has been proposed. The Royal
College of General Practitioners (13) has reviewed
the opportunities for prevention in primary care and
has noted that although much could be done using
existing skills, it considers that resources are
insufficient. Reference has already been made to the
opportunities in primary care that exist for
pharmacists, nurses, volunteers and all concerned
with community development.

Community surveys (14) in the United Kingdom
have shown that the public perceive the general
practitioner as the prime source of advice on health
although it is accepted that their expectations are
not always fulfilled. Clearly the general
practitioner and the members of the primary care team
are key figures in any new initiatives in promoting
health, and the challenge must be to those
professionals to seek new ways of living and working
together to produce a health service more directly
related to the needs of the community, with the
opportunity for active participation by members of
the community in all aspects of health, health
services and social policy relevant to health. As
Tudor Hart (15) points out "The general practitioner
should not only be a symptom responder, but also an

active informed guide through the risks, possibilities, probabilities and remaining impossibilities of medical science".

It would be exciting to set up a new health centre, perhaps involving the same pioneer spirit that was responsible for the Peckham Experiment, but using current knowledge and skills, and building on present day attitudes and aspirations. A new partnership between patients and professionals, involving prevention, care and cure, with participation in planning and policy might be developed, bringing together the health concerns of the community and joint action in seeking to solve them. There might be ease of access to a variety of sources of help - a well stocked library, self help groups, differing professional skills and a commitment to promote environmental and occupational health. Such a project might point afresh to the links between environment and health (16,17) and re-emphasize the importance of humanizing the provision of health care. (18)

Rose (19) in a stimulating paper notes the difference between seeking to detect high risk groups that then require action by the individuals concerned and a mass strategy "whose aim is to shift the whole population's distribution of the risk variable". It also points to the need for greater certainty when the remedy is seen as adding an "unnatural factor", whereas the other preventive measure of removing an unnatural factor and restoring "biological normality" may be advocated more readily on the bases of safety and presumed benefit.

It is interesting to be reminded of the dilemmas and the ethical problems in the preventive approach and this should be opened out for wideranging debate - and not as in the past, left to a few professionals.

Kaprio (20), in his examination of primary health care in Europe, notes the complexity of the relationship between health and society.

At its most theoretical, modern thinking about the health of populations places increasing weight on the interrelationships between factors rather than on individual contributions. Health is seen as a function of the whole social system. Thus the contributions made to health by, for example, nutrition, education, the environment (both physical and socio-psychological), and the socio-economic complex of relative poverty do not depend on 'weighting' that can be attributed to these elements individually, but to the degrees of interaction, or synergism between them ... The best way to improve health may be through behavioural and environmental improvements combined into the provision of care.

The primary health care approach "sees health and enhancement of the quality of life as just one element contributing to the whole process of development."

Kickbush (11) considers that "we are witnessing at the moment a basic change in health education approaches" in the European Region of the World Health Organization, and that these are reflected in four main conceptual reorientations:

- from health prescription to health promotion
- from individualistic behaviour modificiation to a systematic public health approach
- from medical orientation to recognition of lay competence
- from authoritative health education to supportive health education

She believes that the more imaginative forms of health education and information that the above strategy requires can be developed along three main lines:

- raising individual competence and knowledge about health and illness, about the body and its functions, about prevention and coping;
- raising competence and knowledge to use the health care system and to understand its functioning;
- raising awareness about social, political and environmental factors that influence health.

EVALUATION AND RESEARCH

As has been stated on a number of occasions throughout this review, there is a virtual absence of good research and evaluative studies. (21-24) Perhaps this reflects the still uncertain nature of the subject and the lack of an academic base.

The principal impetus for the steady growth of the self-care movement has been not so much the demonstrated efficiency of self-care as the

crisis of confidence in professional medicine.
(25)

While there is an urgent need to evaluate, there is
an awareness that conventional methods of evaluation
are not entirely adequate in looking at the effectiveness of self-care activities. Evaluation must
necessarily be linked to the objectives of self-care.
Many of the traditional outcome indicators, such as
measures of morbidity, mortality and disability are
not sensitive enough for non-life threatening
conditions. New measures of perceived health (26)
relating to the quality of life may be more useful
and appropriate. Here the patient is participating in
the evaluation.

In medicine, there has been a renewed emphasis
on epidemiological research and the analysis of the
many factors involved in the causation of our current
health problems. However, there has been a failure to
match epidemiological research with research founded
on the social, behavioural and educational sciences.
Many of the arguments and views put forward in this
book are not supported fully by research and there is
an urgent task to establish multidisciplinary
research which will confirm or refute and evaluate
what is being proposed as a major aspect of health
and health care in the next few years.

HEALTH FOR ALL BY THE YEAR 2000

This presents a challenge to each country to develop
its own appropriate primary care and that this shoud
be based on needs and not existing professional
services. The Declaration of Alma Ata (27) speaks of
developing programmes "in the spirit of self-
reliance and self-determination" and that these in
turn must be based on the ability "to participate,
individually and collectively in the planning and
implementation of health care". While it was
recognized that primary health care is the only
possible means of providing the least health care to
more than 80% of the underserved and unserved
populations living in parts of the developing world,
the search for new methods, new categories of health
worker, and new approaches in health education can
provide a challenge to the developed as well as the
developing countries. Wagner (28) in writing about
his initial scepticism of this programme, notes the
developments involving participation through the
support and encouragement of the World Health

Organization in several countries. He concludes:

> For health is a means – not an end. Health is a
> process through which individuals and
> communities work to achieve their own ends. If
> health professionals, including W.H.O., give
> the responsibility for this process back to the
> people and honour their own integrity through
> technical cooperation, then by the Year 2000, we
> might have health for all – that is, everyone
> involved in their own health process as a 'means
> toward self and community fulfillment'.

THE WAY AHEAD

It is interesting to note that all the examples just
cited involve a variety of partnership arrangements
between public and professional. Can such be
developed through education of both public and
professionals? Along with approaches such as
'community control', 'self-help', 'human rights' and
'democratisation', participation has become a
pervasive and established factor in society today.
Although its practical effects on the traditional
professionally-directed and hierarchially structured
health services may not be radical or immediately
apparent, participation in health is an idea which
has been born and which has taken on a life of its
own. In spite of doubts and opposition, the struggle
for participation will persist until it becomes an
accepted principle of our health care system.

In the past few years, while the authors have
been reviewing the field, international, national
and local organizations have become much more
specific and direct in their pronouncements.

Speaking at the 11th International Conference
on Health Education, held in Tasmania in 1982, Dr
Halfdan Mahler, Director General of the World Health
Organization (29) summed up the present position and
looked to the future.

> The revolutionary Declaration (of Alma Ata)
> will remain a landmark in the history of health.
> And, as well, in the history of health education
> to which it gave a place of prime importance in
> promoting individual and community self-
> reliance and developing people's ability to
> become full partners in health promotion and
> care. Indeed, one major statement in the
> Declaration is the affirmation that people not

only have the <u>right</u> to participate individually
and collectively in the planning and
implementation of their health care: it is also
their <u>duty</u>. And it is <u>our</u> duty to help them
measure up to this task. No longer should the
health services <u>filter down</u> through a number of
layers to <u>'reach</u> the undeserved'. An upward
movement, starting from the people has now been
initiated. Quite true, participation was
already singled out as an essential component of
health progress by an Expert Committee on Health
Education as far back as 1953. But never before
had it assumed such magnitude. In the past,
participation has too often been equated with
the provision of cheap labour for the
construction of a well, a school or a health
centre, while public funds were being used for
building sophisticated hospitals in larger
cities. To me, participation - or more correctly
<u>involvement</u> - is a mental process in which
individuals and communities identify with a
movement and take responsibility, jointly with
health professionals and others concerned, for
decisions and activities. This is distinctly a
process that health education can promote.

NOTES

1.   D.H.S.S. <u>Inequalities in Health: Report of
a Research Working Group</u> London: H.M.S.O., 1980.
2.   Morris JN. Are Health Services Important
to the People'e Health. <u>British Medical Journal</u> 1980;
1: 167-177.
3.   Kronenfield JJ. Self-care as a Panacea for
the Ills of the Health Care System: An Assessment
<u>Social Science and Medicine</u> 1979; 13A: 263-267.
4.   Backett EM. Consumer Detriment in Health.
In <u>Why the Poor Pay More</u> (Ed. Williams F.) London:
National Consumer Council, 1977.
5.   Mahler H. Health - A Demystification of
Medical Technology. <u>Lancet</u> 1975; 2: 829-833.
6.   Kennedy I. <u>The Unmasking of Medicine</u>
London: Allen and Unwin, 1982.
7.   Backett EM. Discussion. <u>World Health Forum</u>
1981; 2: 191-192.
8.   Levin LS. Self-care in Health: Potentials
and Pitfalls. <u>World Helath Forum</u> 1981; 2: 177-184.
9.   Robinson D. Self-help Groups in Primary
Health Care. <u>World Health Forum</u> 1981; 2: 185-191.
10.   Godber Sir George. Don't Blame the Doctors

- Change the Laws. World Medicine 1981; 16: 17.
11. Kickbush I. Involvement in Health: A Social Concept of Health Education. International Journal of Health Education 181; 24: 3-15.
12. Godber Sir George. Prevention Versus Cure: A Modern Fallacy. World Medicine 1978; No 9: 22-23.
13. Report of a Working Party. Health and Prevention in Primary Care Report from General Practice 18. London: R.C.G.P., 1981.
14. Budd J. and McCron R. The Role of the Mass Media in Health Education. A Report prepared for the Health Education Council Centre for Mass Communications Research. University of Leicester, 1982.
15. Hart JT. Measurement of Omission. British Medical Journal 1982; 284: 1686-1689.
16. Dubos R. Man, Medicine and Environment London: Pall Mall Press, 1968.
17. Dubos R. Man Adapting New Haven: Yale University Press, 1965.
18. Howard J., Davis F., Pope C. and Ruzek A. Humanizing Health Care: The Implications of Technology, Centralization and Self-Care. Medical Care 1977; 15 No 5: Supplement, 11-26.
19. Rose G. Strategy of Prevention: Lessons from Cardiovascular Disease. British Medical Journal 1981; 282: 1847-1857.
20. Kaprio LA. Primary Health Care: Report of the International Conference on Primary Care Copenhagen, W.H.O., 1981.
21. Green LW., Kreuter MW., Deeds SG. and Partridge KB. Health Education Planning. A Diagnostic Approach Palo Alto: Mayfield Publishing Co., 1980.
22. Gunaratne VTH. Health for all by the Year 2000: The Role of Health Education. International Journal of Health Education 1980; 23: Supplement, 1-11.
23. Gross D. and O'Rourke TW. Research and the Future of Health Education. The Journal of School Health 1975; 45: 30-32.
24. Fisher LA. Effectiveness and Efficiency in Health Education Health Economics Research Unit Discussion Paper 09/80. University of Aberdeen: Economics Research Unit, 1980.
25. Martini C. Discussion. World Health Forum 1981; 2: 197-198.
26. Hunt SM. and McEwen J. The Development of A Subjective Health Indicator. Sociology of Health and Illness 1980; 2: 231-246.
27. Report of the International Conference on

Primary Health Care. Declaration of Alma Ata W.H.O./U.N.I.C.E.F., ICPHC/ALA/78. Geneva: World Health Organization, 1978.

28. Wagner MG. The World Health Organization and the Lay Component of Health Care. Medical Sociology News 1980; 7 No 3: 27-30.

29. Mahler H. The New Look in Health Education. The Journal of the Institute of Health Education 1982; 20: No 3: 5-12.

INDEX

abortion 126, 128, 131
Adams 53
addiction 233
advertising 187
Age Concern 169, 227
alternative(s) 20, 145, 169, 230
analgesics 60
Anderson 179
Annas 178
Australia 97, 240

Backett 250, 251
Balding 156
Ballance 234
Baric 142
Bates 97
B.B.C. 152, 154
Bean 114
Bell 55, 56, 59-62
Bender 111-114, 122
Bennett 217
bereaved 228
Berkanovic 142
Black 27
Blum 62
B.M.A. 92, 96, 167, 231
Boyle 179
Braithwaite 188
Brooke 55
Byrne 179
Canada 99
Care 8, 11, 251
  anticipatory 89, 137
  community 12, 227
  health 51, 72-88, 249

primary 55, 57, 88, 92, 101, 193, 196, 214, 220, 240, 251, 252, 254
  terminal 93
career 41
Carlson 9
Cartwright 55, 58-60, 64, 65, 70, 179, 188
Castonquay 19,
categories 112-114
Chadwick 6
change social 7, 10, 15, 174, 239
Channel Four 154
chemist 60, 61
China 128, 140, 141
chiropracter 240
Christopher 60, 61, 68
city inner 250
Claflin 24
classification 112, 115
collective 151
communication 100, 145, 178-180, 186, 191-193
community 8, 10, 55, 87, 90, 125, 140, 141, 148, 193, 213, 215, 218, 235, 238, 252
  action 12
  development 251
  health councils 19, 92, 100, 169
  rural 5
complaints 178
compliance 64, 71, 143, 145, 180, 181, 186

259